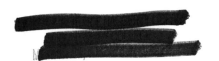

D1565783

Springer Series on Lifestyles and Issues in Aging

Bernard D. Starr, PhD, Series Editor
Marymount Manhattan College, New York, NY

Advisory Board: Robert C. Atchley, PhD; M. Powell Lawton (deceased), PhD; Marjorie H. Cantor, PhD (Hon); Harvey L. Sterns, PhD

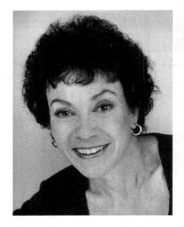

Carole B. Cox, PhD, is Professor at the Graduate School of Social Service, Fordham University. Her gerontological interests and research include the areas of ethnicity and aging, caregiving, and service utilization by older persons and their families. Her research also includes international comparisons of social policy, particularly in the area of community care. Stemming from her work with custodial grandparents, she has written extensively on the issues affecting them and the policies and services that they need in order to carry out their roles. Dr. Cox is the author of numerous articles and book chapters dealing with many aspects of aging. Her previous books include *Home Care: An International Perspective* (coauthor, Abraham Monk), *The Frail Elderly: Problems, Needs, and Community Responses, Ethnicity and Social Work Practice* (coauthor, Paul Ephross), and *Empowering Grandparents Raising Grandchildren: A Training Manual for Group Leaders.* She is also editor of *To Grandmother's House We Go and Stay: Perspectives on Custodial Grandparents.* Dr. Cox is a Fellow of the Gerontological Society of America.

Community Care
for an Aging Society

Issues, Policies, and Services

Carole B. Cox, PhD

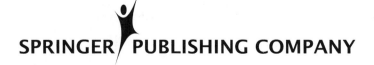

SPRINGER PUBLISHING COMPANY

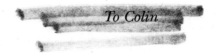
To Colin

Springer Publishing Company, Inc.
11 W 42nd Street
New York, NY 10036-8002

Acquisitions Editor: Helvi Gold
Production Editor: Betsy Day
Cover design by Joanne Honigman

06 07 08 09 / 5 4 3 2

Library of Congress Cataloging-in-Publication Data

Cox, Carole B.
  Community care for an aging society : issues, policies, and services / Carole B. Cox.
    p. cm. — (Springer series on lifestyles and issues in aging)
    Includes bibliographical references and index.
    ISBN 0-8261-2804-1 (alk. paper)
    1. Older people—Care United States. 2. Older people—Services for United States. 3. Community health services for older people—United States.
    I. Title. II. Series: Springer series on the life styles and issues in aging.
HV1461.C739 2005
362.6'0973—dc22   2004024860

Printed in the United States of America by Maple-Vail Book Manufacturing Group.

Contents

Preface

As the new century unfolds, it promises to be composed of a new population. In the next 30 years the number of older adults is expected to double, imposing new challenges and demands on society. With continued improvements in medical care and knowledge of the multitude of factors contributing to a long life, this population of older persons will be healthier and less impaired than earlier cohorts. However, the sheer expansion of the older population and their greater longevity suggests that at any one time there will be significant numbers in need of some care in order to continue living in the community.

Older persons requiring care are often at risk of not having their needs appropriately met when living in the community. Dependency can conflict with an individual's rights of autonomy and self-determination when the types and provision of assistance desired are not available. Families, who provide the majority of assistance, may find themselves unable to meet the needs of their older relatives when support services are unavailable or inaccessible. Consequently, with limited options, seniors needing assistance may find it available only in an institutional setting.

Our present care system continues to maintain a bias toward institutionalization for persons having difficulties functioning on their own. At the same time, most older persons are anxious to remain in the community and in their own homes as long as possible. This overriding interest, concomitant with the immense costs that nursing homes make on public funds, has stimulated interest in community care services as alternatives to institutions. Consequently, both humanitarian and economic forces are working together to make community care a reality for older Americans.

Policies and services are beginning to focus on the community rather than institutions as the primary axis for care. Attention is being given to the needs of older persons and the many options that can help them to remain in the community. Policies and programs at both the federal and local levels, often with the involvement of private foundations and initiatives, are developing and being implemented throughout the country. As these continue to expand, they may serve as important models for the further development of community care in the 21st century.

This book begins by examining the many factors contributing to care needs among older persons, as well as the ways in which impairments are defined and responded to both by the individual and society. Policies and the services enacting them that are essential for enabling older persons to continue to live in the community are addressed in depth. The book describes many of the community care innovations that are in their beginning stages, but which hold the promise of making significant contributions to the well-being and independence of the older population.

Whereas most books on aging tend to focus on either practice or policy issues, this book differs in that both are examined along with their effects on the older population. This offers a greater perspective for understanding needs and the ways in which they are being met. The scope of the book makes it particularly appropriate to students in many disciplines, including gerontology, public policy, social work, sociology, and political science. In addition, the book has practical application for planners and service providers as they focus on designing and implementing policies and programs for older persons.

The needs of the older population and the issues that face us in the 21st century are complex. It is my hope that this book will serve as a springboard for ideas and further discussion on the immense subject of community care. Addressing the challenge now, at the start of the century, is crucial for assuring options for coming generations and ourselves.

Community Care
for an Aging Society

A merica is aging rapidly, with both the proportion and the sheer number of persons 65 and older relative to the rest of the population continuing to increase. Data from the 2000 Census indicate that there are 35 million persons in the United States age 65 and over, accounting for almost 13% of the population. By the year 2030, this number is expected to double to 70 million persons, with the population 85 and over growing faster than any other age group.

Although the functional status of older persons has been improving, with fewer persons reporting limitations (Freedman & Martin, 1998; Waidman & Liu, 2000), the increasing size of the older population, advances in health care, and longer life expectancies suggest there will be no decline in the number of persons needing care. In fact, it's estimated the number of older persons with disabilities will triple between 1985 and 2020 (Manton, Stollard, & Corder, 1998). In addition, there is little evidence of any decrease in the total years that older persons spend disabled (Harper & Forbes, 1998). Consequently, persons may be expected to live many years with a disability and with prolonged needs for assistance.

Providing this care in the most humane and least restrictive environment through a system that offers community options that permit people to remain as independent as possible remains a major social challenge. As the majority of older people desire to remain in their own homes as long as possible and with the costs of institutional care rapidly increasing, new and more expansive systems and models of care are essential. Efforts to develop and implement such models are being carried out by both the public and private sectors throughout the country as communities have begun wrestling with demands of their older citizens. This book examines the many factors that contribute to needs for care as well as the policies and services that are beginning to provide for these needs.

NEEDS FOR CARE

Needs for care among the elderly are primarily associated with physical and functional limitations that affect their ability to care for themselves and increase their dependence on others for assistance. In 2000 just over one quarter, 26.1%, of persons age 65–74 reported a limitation caused by a chronic condition, compared with almost half, 45.1%, of those 75 years and over, and almost three fourths (73.6%) of those 80 and over (Administration on Aging, 2002). Needs for assistance also increase dramatically with age with more than a third of persons over 80 requiring some assistance, in comparison to only 8% of persons with disabilities between the ages of 65 and 69.

In addition, levels of functioning and needs for care are not constant throughout the population. Older persons with higher levels of educa-tion maintain the highest levels of functioning (Manton, Stallard, & Corder, 1997) while higher proportions of women, Blacks, the old-old, and unmarried persons are classified as disabled (Laditka & Jenkins, 2001). Consequently, those with the least resources are likely to have the greatest needs for assistance.

In order to understand and predict needs of care, it is important to have some knowledge of the progression of impairments and the ways in which they impact on the independence and functioning of older persons. Disability has been described as occurring along a specific progression with difficulties occurring in the following order: walking, bathing, transferring, dressing, toileting, feeding (Dunlop, Hughes, & Manheim, 1997), with women spending more time than men in a disabled state.

According to Nagi (1991) people experience functional limitations when they have an impairment that impedes their ability to perform tasks and obligations associated with their usual roles and activities. The Institute of Medicine (1991) builds on this definition by adding risk factors and quality of life measures to the process. These include biologi-cal, social, physical, behavioral, and lifestyle characteristics that affect a person's ability to cope and function.

Further refinement of this model of disability stresses the role of the interaction between the person and the environment as defining the disability that the person experiences (Brandt & Pope, 1997). If a person with a particular limitation has sufficient supports, the impact of a specific disability will not necessarily limit functioning. Consequently, disability is a relative rather than constant concept, since interventions could be used to restore or improve the functioning of an older person.

PHYSICAL CONDITIONS AND IMPAIRMENT

According to the 1990 Survey of Incomes and Program Participation (SIPP), a national survey of the noninstitutionalized population, the major causes of disability for persons 65 and over are arthritis, coronary heart disease, back problems, respiratory conditions, visual impairments, stiffness, and stroke. The major conditions causing persons in the community to require care and assistance are arthritis, coronary heart disease, visual impairments, stroke, and respiratory conditions. In addition, vision and hearing loss exacerbate other impairments (Kempen, Verbrugge, Merrill, & Ormel, 1998; Wallhagen, Strawbridge, Shema, Kurata, & Kaplan, 2001) and the ability to carry out activities of daily living.

For older persons, arthritis and visual impairments, nonfatal conditions, have as much of an impact on limiting activities as fatal conditions such as heart disease, pulmonary disease, and cancer (Verbrugge & Patrick, 1995). The importance of arthritis as a factor in functional limitation is related to its severity (Guccione, Felson, & Anderson, 1990). Persons disabled as a result of the disease are more disabled than others but, at the same time, these disabilities are less severe, have shorter durations, and develop more gradually than disabilities due to other conditions (Verbrugge & Juarez, 2001). Researchers (Boult, Altmann, Gilbertson, Yu, & Kane, 1996) also believe, however, that if the prevalence of arthritis could be reduced by 1% every 2 years, there would be a much greater reduction in functional limitation between the years 2000 and 2049 than would occur by decreasing any other condition by the same amount.

Falls are one of the major causes of disability among older persons. Multiple factors leading to falls include lower extremity weakness, poor grip strength, balance disorders, functional and cognitive impairment, multiple medications, and environmental hazards. Falls have both physical and social consequences, as they can not only cause injury but may also lead to fears and anxiety that can result in loss of self-confidence and in self-imposed limitations on personal functioning. The consequences associated with falling and the fear of falling can contribute significantly to functional decline, and consequently, to increased needs for care.

MENTAL HEALTH

Cognitive Impairment

Cognitive impairment is also a major factor contributing to dependence and care needs among older persons. Although there are several causes of cognitive impairment, Alzheimer's disease (AD) is the most common among older persons. The disease entails a progressive deterioration in the brain that severely jeopardizes a person's ability for self-care. Although it can afflict younger persons, it is most prevalent in the older population, with persons over 85 years of age more than twice as likely to be afflicted.

The course of the disease generally begins with memory loss and some difficulty in performing usual activities such as balancing a checkbook, shopping, or driving. As the illness progresses and the connections between nerve cells in the brain deteriorate, persons lose the abilities to perform most tasks associated with independent functioning, such as dressing, bathing, and feeding oneself, while in the final stage they become bedridden and totally dependent. Indeed, research has indicated that dementia and cognitive impairment are the strongest contributors to functional dependence among the elderly (Aquero-Torres, Fratiglioni, Guo, Viitanen, von Strauss, & Winblad, 1998).

It is estimated that more that 4 million people have AD, with the prevalence rate doubling every 5 years beyond age 65. Estimates are that approximately 360,000 new cases will occur each year and that this number will increase as the population ages (Brookmeyer, Gray, & Kawas, 1998). The extent of the problem in providing care for this population is vividly underscored by its annual costs, which are estimated to be over $100 billion per year (Meek, McKeithan, & Schumock, 1998). Thus, AD and the loss of functioning that it entails are major contributors to the needs for care presented by an aging population.

Mental Illness

Physical impairments are not the only risk factors with regard to impaired functioning among the elderly. Attention must also be paid to the impact of mental health problems, particularly depression, the most prevalent mental illness of the elderly, on the functioning of older adults. According to one estimate, the number of older persons with psychiatric disorders will grow to 13 million persons in the next 3 decades (Jeste et al., 1999).

Data from the Health and Retirement Study (1998) showed depression to be common among older persons, with severe symptoms reported by 15% of those 65 to 69 and by 21% of those 80 to 84, increasing to 34% of persons 85 or older. A study of older persons living in the community found that 19% had 6 or more depressive symptoms and that these were associated with poor self-rated health, disability days, limitations in physical functioning, perceived poor social support, and the use of psychotropic drugs (Hybels, Blazer, & Pieper, 2001).

Other research shows that depressive symptoms among the elderly are prevalent and associated with morbidity and functional impairment (Lyness, King, Cox, Yoediono, & Caine, 1999). Findings from a survey of physical functioning in over 11,000 patients showed that depression strongly affected the ability of the older patient to carry out the activities of daily living (Wells et al., 1989). The disabling effects of depression on bathing, climbing stairs, dressing, socializing, walking, and working were comparable with those of a serious heart condition and greater than those most of the chronic conditions of angina, arthritis, back problems, coronary artery disease, diabetes, gastrointestinal problems, hypertension, and lung problems. The apathy, indecisiveness, withdrawal, and sense of helplessness associated with depression can be conducive to dependency and impaired functioning, as the symptoms affect the older individual's motivation and capacity for self-care.

Depressed elderly engage in less physical activity and have fewer social contacts, which may increase their risk for disability (Pennix, Leveille, Ferrucci, van Eijk, & Guralnik, 1999). However, by offering social interactions to depressed elderly and engaging them in social networks, functional declines can be reduced and even the most depressed can be assisted to maintain their basic functional abilities (Hays, Steffens, Flint, Bosworth, '& George, 2001). Consequently, efforts that address mental health needs of seniors, particularly with regard to reducing their isolation, can be an important factor in strengthening their functional status.

HEALTH CARE

Being able to function in the community may depend a great deal upon the health services available and accessible to the older person with a disability. Health care for the functionally disabled involves both acute and long-term care services and thus requires medical professionals who are knowledgeable about geriatric care. Persons over the age of 65, though they accounted for only 12% of the total population in the year 2000, made 24.3% of all visits to physician offices, according to the National Center for Health Statistics, with almost half of these visits being made to primary care physicians.

Given that the prevalence of chronic illness increases with age, these primary care physicians play a pivotal role in the course of care of these older adults. Unlike acute care, the needs of those with chronic conditions resulting in physical limitations often require the physician to be cognizant of the array of long-term care services to meet these patients' needs. Being able to assess needs and limitations and being knowledgeable about the types of services that can assist the person in the community, ranging from home care to day care and respite care for families is essential if care needs are to be effectively met.

Medicare, the primary health care health care provider for those over 65, is not focused on chronic care needs. According to the National Chronic Care Consortium (2003), elderly with two or more chronic conditions account for 95% of Medicare costs, but current payment plans are not conducive to physicians serving these needs. In addition, there is a paucity of physicians trained in geriatric care. Health problems can be overlooked, dismissed as a normal part of aging, or misdiagnosed, with the consequence being that interventions that could improve these conditions and subsequent functioning are not offered. In addition, the complexity of care required by the frail older adult and the efforts needed to make appropriate assessments, restore functioning, and even arrange for and coordinate services demand extensive planning and time. To date, Medicare does not reimburse physicians for the time it takes to provide the types of care management that these persons require.

The demands that those with chronic disabilities are placing on the health care system are not going unrecognized. The Geriatric Care Act of 2003 would authorize Medicare coverage of assessment and care coordination of those with serious and disabling chronic conditions. The proposed legislation would also expand medical residency training in geriatrics so as to engage and develop a more knowledgeable and skilled cadre of physicians to serve this population. The act underscores the important role played by families of the frail as it includes support for both patient and family education and counseling as well as the development of self-management services.

MENTAL HEALTH CARE

With mental health playing such a key role in the functioning of older adults, detection and treatment of the illnesses and disorders that can impede functioning should be an urgent concern. Unfortunately, older people are the most at risk of not receiving mental health care, and the least likely to visit mental health professionals.

Less than 3% of persons over the age of 65 receive outpatient mental health treatment from a specialist, a rate that is much lower than any other age group (Olfson & Pincus, 1996). When persons do go for care, they tend to seek help from their primary care providers who may or may not detect their problems. A vivid illustration of the impact of inadequate treatment is found in a study of suicide among older adults (Conwell, 1994). Twenty percent had visited a physician the day of their suicide, 40% within the week, and 70% within 1 month of the suicide.

Feelings of stigma associated with mental health problems, issues associated with access, financing and insurance, feelings of denial, and an absence of trained mental health professionals are among the reasons for the under-treatment of these conditions. In addition, although available, appropriate treatments and interventions that can relieve symptoms and improve functioning are not being fully implemented in clinical practice (Bartels & Smyer, 2002).

A shortage of trained professionals and limited payments and reimbursement for community mental health care are two of the major impediments to service. With Medicare, patients are required to pay 50% of the costs of outpatient mental health visits, in comparison with 20% of other physician visits. With limited prescription drug coverage by Medicare and many other insurance plans, pharmacological treatments for depression and other mental illness are often inaccessible to many older persons.

RISKS FOR IMPAIRMENT AND CARE

As we enter the 21st century, major advances in health care and in our understanding of the nature and progress of disabilities can help to prevent or delay functional dependency among the older population. Moreover, new technologies, methods of rehabilitation, and services, coupled with alterations in a person's environment, can negate many of the consequences associated with disability and limited functioning and thus increase the potential of preventing dependency. Equally important is the role that psychosocial resources—including one's own sense of mastery and control, and personal relationships—have in improving functioning and helping persons to cope better with chronic conditions and disabilities.

Findings from a large-scale longitudinal study of aging indicate that risks for functional decline, even among older adults with chronic conditions, can be influenced by physical exercise, social support, self-efficacy beliefs, and feelings of psychological well-being (Seeman & Chen, 2002). Having emotional support may be protective of decline as it enables persons to better deal with the stress that can accompany functional limitations and chronic conditions.

One of the main precursors of dependency in older adults is a sedentary lifestyle. Decreased physical activity leads to muscle weakness and bone fragility, and older persons generally move less frequently than younger persons. In a comprehensive review of the concept of frailty in older adults, Bortz (2002) describes it as a state of muscular weakness with other secondary losses in function and structure that are usually initiated by decreased levels of physical activity. Lifestyle interventions, including changes in nutrition and physical activity, may play major roles in preventing disability and functional loss among older persons.

Maintaining muscle strength is fundamental to performance of many of the tasks of daily living, such as getting out of bed, walking, or rising from a chair. In addition, weakness in the lower body and impaired strength increase the risk of falling and of being injured as a result of a fall (Work, 1989). Although the evidence is still inconclusive, there is some which suggests that exercise and weight-bearing exercises can be important factors in reducing falls among the elderly and thus in reducing the risk of serious disability.

Sedentary lifestyles also lead to a more rapid decrease in leg muscles. Exercise programs continued over time can counteract this decrease by increasing muscle mass and bone density. Intervention studies using exercise programs for frail older adults demonstrate significant improvement in the subjects' balance, muscle strength, walking function, and self-assessed functional ability (Worm et al., 2001). Of particular importance are exercises that increase strength by increasing muscle mass. Even the oldest of the old, those 85 and over, have been found to significantly increase their strength through weight lifting exercises (Shephard, 1987). According to Shephard, participation by the elderly in three 1-hour exercise classes per week may reduce health care costs of acute and chronic treatment, mental health treatment, and extended residential care by more than $600 per year for each older person.

Health education activities, as they focus on functioning and positive health practices, can counteract belief systems and attitudes viewing dependency and frailty as unavoidable risks, even for those with impairments. Studies show that older persons who lead healthy lifestyles and engage in activities that promote their health are functionally more healthy than their peers (Duffy & MacDonald,1990). Moreover, the same data found that the oldest and most impaired group, those 85 and older, had the highest exercise levels, providing further support that functioning is not necessarily equated with impairment.

The prevention of mental impairments leading to dependency is potentially even more complex than that associated with the prevention of physical ones. At the same time, as many spheres of the older individuals' lives may contribute to their mental health, there are innumerable areas for intervention. Socialization programs, environmental supports, therapy, and counseling are examples of interventions that can assist persons dealing with both physical and emotional loss and transitions. The availability of these programs and services, tailored to the needs of specific groups, can be significant in helping persons adjust to and cope with the many transitions incumbent in aging.

THEORETICAL PERSPECTIVES ON IMPAIRMENT AND CARE

This review of the factors conducive to functional impairment and consequent needs for care among older persons underscores the interactions and complexity of factors that affect the well-being and status of the older population. Many theories of social gerontology can assist in unraveling this complexity by providing a conceptual framework linking these factors together in a coherent manner. These theories can also indicate those who are most vulnerable to dependency as well as providing a framework for the development of specific interventions.

Continuity theory is particularly pertinent to the experience of older adults at risk of functional declines. This theory maintains that older persons seek to continue in their usual roles and lifestyles throughout the aging process. Individuals have a coherent structure that persists over time but allows for a variety of changes to occur (Atchley, 1989).

Two fundamental aspects of the theory are internal and external continuity. Internal continuity refers to the persistence of ideas, personality, preferences, and temperament. People seek to maintain a sense of internal continuity because it offers a sense of competence, control, and self-esteem.

External continuity refers to the maintenance of social roles, role relationships, and activities. External continuity is important to the maintenance of strong social supports, and perhaps more significantly, to the maintenance of a strong self-concept. Internal continuity appears to remain constant over time, in that persons tend to interact with those who support their sense of self and who maintain their sameness. A desire for external continuity also appears to be the norm in that persons continue to use established skills, perform accustomed activities, and interact within the same relationships.

However, both mental and physical impairments can pose obstacles to continuity. The older person whose memory is no longer intact will be thwarted in his or her attempt to maintain internal continuity. The person with physical impairments that make the performance of traditional skills impossible may find external continuity jeopardized. In both cases, reductions in social support systems can further threaten continuity. Unfortunately, such transitions in these systems frequently occur simultaneously with the older person's impairments, so that discontinuity develops. It is with this discontinuity that the older individual becomes susceptible to a decline in functioning.

According to symbolic interaction theory, identity is developed and maintained through interactions and reinforcement with others in society (Mead, 1934). Reference groups, those with whom the individual identifies, and significant others, those who are influential in the individual's life, are key actors in the development of self. Through interactions with these sets, proper roles and expected behaviors are learned and self-concept is developed.

As applied to older persons with impaired functioning, they are susceptible to developing a negative self-concept due to the nature of their interactions with others. As others perceive and treat older persons as dependent, through actions and behaviors that reinforce their limitations, they become increasingly susceptible to defining themselves as frail and in need of care. Accordingly, they may begin to further limit their activities and question their own self-sufficiency. Dependency is therefore socially construed as it becomes a part of the individual's self identity.

"Learned helplessness" builds upon symbolic interaction theory and can give further insight into the onset of dependency. According to the concept, helplessness develops as the impaired begin to accept the loss of control over their own lives and their dependency. Individuals become increasingly passive, dependent, and helpless, and begin to lose confidence in their ability to function (Seligman, 1975). Unfortunately, others, as they offer assistance, only serve to exacerbate this negative self-concept. Rather than focusing on strengths, they tend to focus on the disability with the result being that the disabled elderly perceive themselves as helpless and dependent on others.

The interactionist perspective is further delineated in the theory of social breakdown/reconstruction (Bengtson, 1976). The theory delineates many factors in the environment that can act to threaten and destroy the older person's sense of competence. As abilities become less acute, the impaired individual is vulnerable to being labeled dependent with the identity reinforced by those offering care and assistance.

The outcome is that as care is accepted, the older person is vulnerable to becoming increasingly dependent.

Using a reconstructionist model, Bengtson proposes that the vicious circle leading to dependency can be broken. By having those offering care and support reinforcing the strengths and coping abilities of the older person, confidence can be rebuilt and breakdown halted or reversed. In this way dependency does not become a part of the identity and functioning may be at least partially restored.

Ecological models which focus on persons in the environment are particularly appropriate to the functioning and care requirement of older adults, as they can help identify those areas where supports that can enhance functioning are needed. Lawton and Nahemow's (1973) model of environmental press is based on a balance point between environmental demands and individual capabilities, with optimal functioning occurring when the older person is able to satisfy behavioral needs and maintain psychological well-being. If the relationship changes so that the environmental pressures become too severe or the person's competency to deal with the environment is weakened, interventions that modify or alter either the setting or the capability of the person are required. In addition, the individual's own appraisal of the situation is an important factor in determining press, as it affects whether or not they believe a disability exists or what action to take to moderate it (Lawton, 1998).

These theories suggest that individual needs for care, in addition to stemming from functional impairments, can be affected by social-psychological factors and that disability or impairment is not necessarily sufficient as a predictor. A devalued self-image associated with a sense of helplessness that is reinforced by others can contribute to the development or enhancement of dependency and hence the needs for care. In addition, as the environment fails to respond to the abilities of the older person, persons become increasingly vulnerable.

In addition to theories that focus on individual responses to aging and impairment, an important framework for examining the functioning and status of older persons in a society is the political economy perspective. This perspective views old age and the problems associated with aging as socially constructed and resulting from the unequal distribution of resources. The central focus is on analyzing the structural conditions and socioeconomic factors that create inequality in old age and affect the policy interventions that occur in a capitalist society.

Using a political economy perspective, the challenge is not to see how persons interpret their private troubles but to see how these private troubles become public issues (Estes, Gerard, Zones, & Swan, 1984).

The perspective helps to explain the experience of old age, the patterns of inequality among older people, and how public policy may ameliorate or exacerbate such inequalities (Quadagno & Reid, 1999).

Consequently, the political economy framework expands our understanding of the ways in which society offers resources and care to older adults. By examining the impact that class divisions, gender, and discrimination have had on persons throughout their lives and the ways in which services have been offered or available to them, a greater knowledge of the process of current provisions to older persons can be obtained. The perspective highlights the inequalities in society, their impact on the older population, and the ways in which social policy can continue to perpetuate such inequalities.

CONSEQUENCES OF IMPAIRMENT

Functional impairment can limit a person's autonomy because it commonly involves restrictions in the individual's capacity for decision making. Older adults who require assistance either from their family or from agencies frequently find that the number of choices regarding their care is limited as a consequence of their impairments. In many instances, dependency upon others means giving these persons the power of decision making in their lives.

Losing the autonomy of action and the ability to function independently is often associated with forfeiting the capacity for self-actualization. Dependency can connote that the person no longer has the ability to act with any judgment. Consequently, by requiring care, a person can be placed at risk of having decision-making powers revoked or restricted due to perceived incompetence. Obviously, these perceptions can further threaten the individual's self concept and eventual ability to remain independent.

As dependency can convey vulnerability, it can threaten a person's right to autonomy and self-determination. As policies, families, friends, and services wrestle with meeting the care needs of older persons, they are often at risk of infringing on their basic political and social rights. Planning and designing appropriate services and interventions that address their needs in the community without creating further dependency or inequality is therefore an expansive task that necessitates sensitivity and commitment.

The consequences of requiring care are not restricted to older persons themselves, as it is families that continue to provide the majority of this assistance. The challenges and burdens that these caregivers encounter have been well documented. Thus, although relatives are the foundation for community care, this is not without consequence to their own well-being. In addition, the continued availability of these family caregivers is debatable. Shifts in the demographics of the population mean fewer adult children are available to care for the burgeoning number of elderly, while spousal caregivers are likely to be elderly themselves, affecting the extent and types of care that they can provide.

Finally, it is important to remember that growing old does not necessitate disability and frailty, and healthy aging is not an oxymoron. The majority of the elderly reside in the community and function with little restriction on their activities, and even when restricted, are able to maintain their independence. At the same time, the rapid growth of the older population means there will be increasing numbers of persons with chronic illness and functional limitations who will require some assistance in order to live as they would desire. The continuing challenge is to ensure that older persons have options with regard to resources and services that can enable them to remain as autonomous as possible, in a supportive environment with a high quality of life.

SUMMARY

This book addresses some of the major issues confronting the frail elderly. As this introduction indicates, frailty cannot be narrowly defined or predicted. Many factors, physical, mental, and social can result in frailty and thus appropriate interventions must be made in accordance with this diversity of causes. The majority of the those with impairments reside in the community and therefore the focus of this book is on the ways in which the community responds to the problems and needs of this population.

Impairment and disability are not going to disappear, nor are the demands and needs of those requiring care and desiring to remain in the community. With the expansion of the elderly population, it becomes increasingly important to understand who is most at risk of frailty, and why. Only with such knowledge can a comprehensive framework of policies and services directed at both prevention and care be designed.

The ramifications of an aging population and of the needs of those with functional limitations affect everyone and defy simple unitary solutions. The issues surrounding such care are broad, involving many spheres of life. In order for responses to be effective they must extend beyond just one field so that they can best encompass the many variables influencing well-being and independence in later life.

This book, as it addresses the issue of frailty among elderly in the community, begins, in chapter 2, with a discussion of the way in which frailty is defined and the complexity of the term itself. Policy provides a necessary framework for meeting the needs of the frail, and as the book describes in chapter 3, these policies are being designed at many levels, federal, state, and local, yet their effectiveness remains questionable. The community responds to the needs of the impaired elderly through services offered through both the public and private sectors. Chapter 4 describes the major services that can have an impact on the lives of these elderly. Housing for older persons with impairments remains an overriding concern, and in chapter 5 the various available options, including adaptations in the home, are described.

Families provide the bulwark of assistance to these elderly. Chapter 6 presents theoretical perspectives for understanding the involvement of these family caregivers while also discussing the extent of family involvement, its effects on the older person, and its effects on the caregiver. As ethnicity and minority group membership in particular can influence both the development and perception of frailty, as well as the way in which the family responds to it, chapter 7 is devoted to an elaboration of this subject.

Much innovation is occurring throughout this country with regard to the care of older persons in the community. Chapter 8 describes some of these innovations as they may provide important models for programs and services. Chapter 9 is an attempt to summarize and draw conclusions about the needs of this population and the effectiveness of current responses, and suggests recommendations for change.

REFERENCES

Administration on Aging. (2002). *A profile of older Americans.* U.S. Department of Health and Human Services. Washington, DC: Administration on Aging.

Aquero-Torres, H., Fratiglioni, L., Guo, Z., Vittanen, M., von Strauss, E., & Winblad, G. (1998). Dementia is the major cause of functional dependence in the elderly: 3-year follow-up data from a population based study. *American Journal of Public Health, 88,* 1452–1456.

Atchley, R. C. (1989). A continuity theory of normal aging. *Gerontologist, 29,* 183–190.

Bartels, S., & Smyer, M. (2002). Mental disorders of aging: An emerging public health crisis. *Generations, 26,* 14–20.

Bengtson, V. (1976). *The social psychology of aging.* Indianapolis: Bobbs Merrilll.

Bortz, W. (2002). A conceptual framework of frailty: A review. *Journal of Gerontology A., Biological and Medical Sciences, 57,* M283–M288.

Boult, C., Altmann, M., Gilbertson, D., Yu, C., & Kane, R. (1996). Decreasing disability in the 21st century: The future effects of controlling six fatal and non-fatal conditions. *American Journal of Public Health, 86,* 1388–1393.

Brandt, E., & Pope, A. (Eds.) (1997). Models of disability and rehabilitation. In E. Brand & A. Pope (Eds.), *Enabling America: Assessing the role of rehabilitation in science and engineering* (pp. 62–80). Washington, DC: National Academy Press.

Brookmeyer, R., Gray, S., & Kawas, C. (1998). Projections of Alzheimer's disease in the United States and the public health impact of delaying disease onset. *American Journal of Public Health, 88,* 1337–1342.

Conwell, Y. (1994). Suicide in elderly patients. In L. Scheider, C. Reynolds, B. Lebowitz, & A. Friedhoff (Eds.), *Diagnosis and treatment of depression in late life* (pp. 397–418). Washington, DC: American Psychiatric Press.

Duffy, M., & MacDonald, E. (1990). Determinants of functional health of older persons. *Gerontologist, 30,* 503–510.

Dunlop, D., Hughes, S., & Manheim, L. (1997). Disability in activities of daily living: Patterns of change and hierarchy of disability. *American Journal of Public Health, 87,* 378–383.

Estes, C., Gerard, L., Zones, J., & Swan, J. (1984). *Political economy, health and aging.* Boston: Little, Brown.

Freedman, V., & Martin, L. (1998). Understanding trends in limitations in older Americans. *American Journal of Public Health, 88,* 1457–1462.

Guccione, A., Felson, D., & Anderson, J. (1990). Defining arthritis and measuring functional status in elders: Methodological issues in the study of disease and physical disability. *American Journal of Public Health, 80,* 90–95.

Harper, D., & Forbes, W. (1998). Aging, health risks, and cumulative disability. *New England Journal of Medicine, 339,* 481–482.

Hays, J., Steffens, D., Flint, E., Bosworth, H., & George, L. (2001). Does social support buffer functional decline in elderly patients with unipolar depression? *American Journal of Psychiatry, 158,* 1850–1855.

Hybels, D., Blazer, D., & Pieper, C. (2001). Towards a threshold for subthreshold depression: An analysis of correlates of depression by severity of symptoms using data from an elderly community sample. *Gerontologist, 41,* 357–365.

Institute of Medicine. (1991). *Disability in America: Towards a national agenda for prevention.* Washington, DC: National Academy Press.

Jeste, D., Alexopoules, G., Bartels, S., Cummings, J., Gallo, J., Gottlieb, G., et al. (1999). Consensus statement on the upcoming crisis in geriatric mental health, research agenda for the next 2 decades. *Archives of General Psychiatry, 56,* 848–853.

Kempen, G., Verbrugge, L., Merrill, S., & Ormel, J. (1998). The impact of multiple impairments on disability in community-dwelling older people. *Age and Aging, 27,* 595–604.

Laditka, J., & Jenkins, C. (2001). Difficulty or dependency? Effects of measurement scales on disability prevalence among older adults. *Journal of Health and Social Policy, 13,* 1–15.

Lawton, M. (1998). Environment and aging: Theory revisited. In R. Scheidt & P. Windley (Eds.), *Empowerment and aging theory: A focus on housing* (pp. 1–13). Westport, CT: Greenwood.

Lawton, M., & Nahemow, I. (1973). Ecology and the aging process. In C. Eisdorfer & M. Lawton (Eds.), *Psychology of adult development and aging* (pp. 619–674). Washington, DC: American Psychological Association.

Lyness, J., King, D., Cox, C., Yoediono, Z., & Caine, E. (1999). The importance of subsyndromal depression in older primary care patients: Prevalence and associated functional disability. *Journal of the American Geriatrics Society, 47,* 647–652.

Manton, K., Stallard, E., & Corder, L. (1997). Education-specific estimates of life expectancy and age-specific disability in the U.S. elderly population, 1982–1991. *Journal of Aging and Health, 9,* 419–450.

Manton, K., Stallard, E., & Corder, L. (1998). The dynamics of dimensions of age-related disability 1992 to 1994 in the U.S. elderly population. *Journal of Gerontology, Biological Sciences, 53A,* B59–B70.

Mead, G. (1934). *Mind, self and society.* Chicago: University of Chicago Press.

Meek, P., McKeithan, K., & Schumock, G. (1998). Economic considerations in Alzheimer's disease. *Pharmacotherapy, 18,* 68–73.

Nagi, S. (1991). Disability concepts revisited: Implications for prevention. In A. Pope & A. Tarlov (Eds.), *Disability in America: Toward a national agenda for prevention* (pp. 304–327). Washington, DC: National Academy Press.

National Chronic Care Consortium. (2003). *Moving to better chronic care in medicine: NRCCC proposals for change.* Washington, DC: Author.

National Institute on Aging. (1998). *The health and retirement study: A longitudinal study of health, retirement, and aging.* Rockville, MD: Author.

Olfson, M., & Pincus, H. (1996). Outpatient mental health care in nonhospital settings: Distribution of patients across provider groups. *American Journal of Psychiatry, 153,* 1353–1356.

Pennix, B., Leveille, S., Ferrucci, L., van Eijk, J., & Guralnik, J. (1999). Exploring the effect of depression on physical disability: Longitudinal evidence from the established population for epidemiologic studies of the elderly. *American Journal. of Public Health, 89,* 1346–1352.

Quadagno, J., & Reid, J. (1999). The political economy perspective in aging. In V. Bengtson & K. Schaie (Eds.), *Handbook of theories of aging* (pp. 344–360). New York: Springer Publishing.

Seeman, T., & Chen, X. (2002). Risk and protective factors for physical functioning in older adults with and without chronic conditions: MacArthur studies of successful aging. *Journal of Gerontology, Social Sciences, 57B,* S135–S144.

Seligman, M. (1975). *Helplessness.* San Francisco: W. H. Freeman.

Shepherd, R. (1987). *Physical activity in aging* (2nd ed.). London: Croom Helm.

Verbrugge, L., & Juarez, L. (2001). Profile of arthritis disability. *Public Health Reports, 116,* Suppl. 1, 157–179.

Verbrugge, L., & Patrick, D. (1995). Seven chronic conditions: Their impact on U.S. adults' activity levels and use of medical services. *American Journal of Public Health, 85,* 173–182.

Waidmann, T., & Liu, K. (2000). Disability trends among elderly persons and implications for the future. *Journal of Gerontology, 55B,* S298–S307.

Wallhagen, W., Strawbridge, M., Shema, S., Kurata, J., & Kaplan, G. (2001). Comparative impact of hearing and vision impairment on subsequent functioning. *Journal of the American Geriatrics Society, 49,* 1086–1092.

Wells, K., Stewart, A., Hays, R., Burman, M., Rogers, W., Daniels, M., Berry, A., Greenfield, S., & Ware, J. (1989). The functioning and well-being of depressed patients—results from the medical outcomes study. *Journal of the American Medical Association, 262,* 914–919.

Work, J. (1989). Strength training: A bridge to independence for the elderly. *Physician and Sports Medicine, 17,* 134–140.

Worm, C., Vad, E., Puggaard, L., Stovring, H., Lauritsen, J., & Kragstrup, J. (2001). Effects of a multicomponent exercise program on functional ability in community-dwelling frail older adults. *Journal of Aging and Physical Activity, 9,* 414–424.

Determining Needs for Care

Eligibility for the majority of public programs and services as well as decisions regarding the capacity of an older individual to remain in the community are generally based on a person's functional ability. Functional limitation pertains to restriction or inability to perform an activity in a manner that is considered normal, resulting from an impairment. Functional limitation increases the risk of disability. Disability is an inability or limitation in performing socially defined activities and roles, such as shopping for groceries (Pope & Tarlov, 1991, p. 79). Disablement is a process, with functional limitation an interim state between impairment and disability (Nagi, 1991). These distinctions become important in the understanding of the disablement process, the design of interventions, and the development of policies to serve persons in differing stages of the course.

Often, the term "frail" is used to identify individuals who have difficulties in functioning. For many programs, the definition of frailty is synonymous with functional impairment, functional dependency, or functional disability. These terms are frequently used interchangeably, most often describing older adults with diminished or declining capacity for independence. An individual may be functionally impaired due to hearing loss, functionally dependent due to an inability to use transportation, and functionally disabled due to a chronic illness such as arthritis which impedes mobility.

FRAILTY

In the early 1970s, as the needs of older adults associated with their functional limitations became more apparent, the Federal Council on Aging drew attention to their concerns, providing one of the first definitions of the term "frail elderly." The frail elderly are "those, usually but not always, over the age of 75, who because of the accumulation of various continuing problems often require one or several supportive services in order to cope with daily life" (U.S. Department of Health, Education, and Welfare, 1978). Frailty was also defined as involving the "loss of a social-support system to the extent that the person is unable to maintain a household or social contacts without continuing assistance from others" (p. 15).

Beginning in the 1970s, the Older Americans Act (1965, amended), the only comprehensive legislative plan for older adults in this country, gave special attention to the frail elderly, categorizing them as a vulnerable group requiring special attention due to having "greatest economic or social need." Social need emphasizes the noneconomic factors— physical and mental disabilities, language barriers, cultural and social isolation, and ethnic or racial status that restrict an individual's ability to perform normal daily tasks or that threaten the capacity to live independently (Coombs, Lambert, & Quirk, 1982).

The World Health Organization defines frailty as "any restriction or lack (resulting from an impairment) of an ability to perform an activity in the manner or within the range considered normal for a human being" (World Health Organization, 1980). Given this very broad interpretation, restriction may be due to any type of impairment and frailty associated with a multitude of causes. Among its many definitions are that it is the result of excess demands imposed upon reduced capacity (Powell, 1997), a diminished capacity to carry out the important practical and social activities of daily living (Brown, Renwick, & Raphael, 1995), or a state that makes persons inherently vulnerable to challenge from the environment (Strawbridge, Shema, Balfour, Higby, & Kaplan, 1998).

The lack of any uniform definition of the term "frailty" is highlighted by the fact that health professionals working with the elderly fail to agree on what the term actually measures (Kaethier, Molnar, Mitchell, Soucie, & Man-Son-Hing, 2003). Although the majority of persons surveyed claimed the term was useful, it is striking that the interpretations ranged from age-induced phenomena to a need for institutional care, with only half of the professionals stating that it is related to function and independence in older adults.

An awareness of the varying connotations of impairment is critical because such definitions are often the criteria for policies and the services whereby they are implemented. Functional status is generally used as an indicator for the need of long-term care services. With the term being so diffuse and amenable to many interpretations, it is not surprising that multiple instruments are used as measures. An underlying concern is that they may be measuring different things.

ACTIVITIES OF DAILY LIVING

The assessment of functional impairment is commonly based upon an older person's ability to perform the activities of daily living (ADLs). These activities are those that are habitually performed and are required for independent living. The ADLs traditionally include bathing, dressing, toileting, transferring between bed and chair, continence, and eating. Presently, there are more than 50 ADL instruments in use measuring functional status.

There are several advantages for using these criteria as assessment measures. They are easy to define, are quantifiable, can be based on self-report, and are sensitive to changes in functioning. Moreover, the measures are easy to administer and can therefore readily be applied to large populations as a screening device, while also being used by paraprofessionals. Instruments measuring ADLs are widely used in surveys examining the functional status of community elderly as well as bases for estimates of the numbers of persons requiring assistance.

Measuring the Activities of Daily Living

Originally developed in the early 1960s, measurements of the ADLs were used as a means of evaluating treatment and assessing the prognosis for aged and chronically ill persons. The Katz Index of Independency (1963) is one of the earliest instruments designed to measure ADLs, originally used to measure functioning among hospitalized patients. This instrument, as well as assessing functional ability in six specific tasks, also scales the ADLs in a hierarchial manner according to the effects of each on independence. Requiring assistance in bathing is less limiting to the individual's independence than being dependent in eating or toileting. Scores for each item are measured according to whether the respondent is independent or dependent. These scores are summed to provide an overall measure of dependency.

The Katz instrument is only one of many used to measure physical functioning. With the growth of the older population and an increase in services, newer instruments aimed at measuring eligibility have been developed. In some instances, these are unique to specific programs and their service goals while others are more widely utilized.

Some of these instruments are restricted to just five ADLs, while others ask about additional activities. These differences, however, are significant in that with more activities being measured there will be an increase in the number of persons who will be classified as "disabled."

But an inherent limitation in all of these scales that assess frailty on the sole basis of physical functioning is that they frequently do not measure the extent of dysfunction or adaptation that the older individual has made to the impairment.

As the use of the ADLs as a criterion for disability has grown, it has been adapted to meet program needs and priorities. As an example, walking was not included in the original list of ADLs since mobility limitation is not consistently associated with dependence. The use of walkers, canes, and even wheelchairs enables impaired elderly to function independently. Walking, therefore, does not fit into the hierarchial pattern of dependency. However, in many instruments, walking is included along with other activities such as going outside or getting around inside the house. An elderly person may be deemed physically fit according to one instrument and functionally impaired on another due to problems with mobility or difficulties in walking on the street.

In measuring the degree of disability, instruments also differ according to whether they assess the degree of difficulty in performing a specific task or whether the activity can be completed with assistance. Some instruments may count a person as dependent only if human assistance is required, while others include mechanical assistance such as grab bars, special beds, or walkers as indicators of dependency. Again, the importance of this difference is more than just semantics, since the more inclusive definition will assess more persons as impaired and thus eligible for assistance. Moreover, measures that are limited to only two response categories, "can or cannot perform," will provide different estimates from those inquiring about the amount of assistance or supervision needed.

To further complicate the issue of measuring impairment, tools also differ with regard to how respondents are asked to define themselves. Some may ask the extent of difficulty encountered in completing a specific task, while others phrase the response categories according to how much assistance is needed. In the one instance, an individual may respond that the activity is completed without any difficulty and fail to mention that this is due to receiving assistance. In the other, the responses may reflect whether a person requires assistance but not whether such assistance is actually available. Moreover, response categories such as "a lot, some, not much, or none" offer much latitude for subjective interpretations.

Differences in the prevalence of disability have been found on whether items measure degree of difficulty in performing a task, or dependency (requiring assistance) in order to complete it (Kovar & Lawton, 1994). Estimates of disability are 1.5 to 4 times higher using the difficulty measure rather than need or dependency (Jette, 1994). Jette also found that older adults with less education or income had more discordance between their needs and available help, meaning that they had a difficulty with an activity but did not have either human or technical assistance to help them. Other studies have found that less advantaged older persons, those with less education, and in particular unmarried women with less education, are the most sensitive to the type of ADL scale, whether it measures difficulty or dependency (Laditka & Jenkins, 2001). Consequently, particular subgroups may be ineligible for services if dependency rather than difficulty is used as the main criterion for services.

Weiner, Hanley, Clark, and Van Nostrand (1990) provide examples of the variation among instruments according to the types of information used to record disability. Among 11 national surveys collecting information on the ADL status of older persons, 3 recorded whether the disability had lasted for a minimum period of time, 4 recorded the level of difficulty in completing a task, and 3 recorded whether or not the person required assistance. All of the 11 instruments asked if the person received human assistance, while 9 out of the 11 asked if the person used special equipment in completing the activity.

An important and often overlooked aspect of impairment is that it is not a constant. It is estimated that at least 50% of impaired elderly alter in their ADLs in a 6-month period (Liu & Cornelius, 1989). Such intense change in status has important ramifications for services and needs for assistance. Instruments, however, do not necessarily measure the duration of the impairment or plan for reassessments. Many only record the older person as functionally impaired if at the time of the interview a difficulty in completing an activity is reported. Other instruments define a limitation in functioning only if the disability has lasted or can be expected to last for 90 days or longer.

Scales also vary in their administration: self-report, proxy-response, and performance measures. Self-report has the older adult describe his or her own functional status, while the proxy measure relies on the perceptions of another individual. When giving self-reports, there is some concern that persons may overestimate their abilities, since proxies generally assess the person's disability higher than self-reports (Spector, 1997). Proxies may also not be informed enough to make accurate assessments and their reports may also be related to the amount of care they provide (Zimmerman & Magaziner, 1994).

Performance scales are formal evaluations of the individual's functioning made by an assessor in a controlled situation. The problems with this approach are the length of the assessment, the training of the rater, the need for special equipment, and the fact the activities are not performed in the older person's own environment (Spector, 1997). Research has also found the relationships between self-reports, interviewer-administered, and performance-based testing to be very weak, suggesting they do not measure the same constructs or abilities (Reuben, Valle, Hays, & Siu, 1995).

In addition, there is concern that little attention is given to distinctions among tenses of functioning (hypothetical, experimental, and enacted), because what people say they can do and what they actually do at home can differ (Glass, 1998). Examples of hypothetical measures are asking the person if they can do a task, if they require assistance, and how much difficulty they have. Experimental measures ask persons to demonstrate their ability in a laboratory or clinic, while enacted measures have the person perform the activities at home. The discrepancies found among the measures suggest that many complex factors affect the older person's ability to function in the home and that these are generally not assessed. Thus, it is not clear why certain older persons may overcome functional limitations while others with low levels of disability may have low levels of function.

INSTRUMENTAL ACTIVITIES OF DAILY LIVING

The instrumental activities of daily living (IADLs) are also used as indicators of impairment and frailty. These activities are tasks commonly done by individuals in the community as a normal part of daily living and are essential for adaptation in the environment. They include using the telephone, shopping, housekeeping, doing laundry, taking medications, using transportation, and managing finances. Unlike the ADLs, these activities measure cognitive as well as physical capacity, and therefore may provide a more comprehensive assessment of the individual. Studies have also shown that IADL impairment is most closely predicted by impairment in the lower body, such as difficulties with walking, standing, crouching, and lifting, than in upper extremity functions, such as grasping or reaching, thus reflecting the importance of movements needed for shopping, housekeeping, and food preparation (Lawrence & Jette, 1996).

Measuring the Instrumental Activities of Daily Living

A frequently used scale for measuring IADLs is one developed by Lawton and Brody (1969). Data are collected from the elderly individual or a caregiver on independence in using the telephone, shopping, food preparation, housekeeping, doing laundry, the use of public transportation, taking medications, and handling finances. Scoring ranges from totally independent in each activity to totally dependent, with item scores measured on an 8-point Guttman scale for women and a 5-point Guttman scale for men. Higher scores reflect greater total dependence.

Instrumental activities of daily living are also measured with the Older Americans Resources and Services (OARS) instrument (Duke University Center for the Study on Aging, 1978). This instrument includes seven items: telephone use, travel, shopping, meal preparation, housework, taking own medications, and handling personal finances. In contrast to the Lawton and Brody scale, all items are asked of both men and women and responses are recorded in only three categories: can be performed unaided; some help is needed; and cannot be performed at all. In order to overcome the bias that might accompany gender-related responses, the items may also be asked "could you perform . . . ?"

Further refinement of this scale suggests that it may be accurately reduced to only five items and still identify elderly individuals in the community who are impaired (Fillenbaum, 1985). Accordingly, the ability to use the telephone and to take own medications are not necessarily predictive of the ability to remain independent in the community. Instead, the items may be reduced to the ability to use transportation, shop, prepare food, do housework, and manage finances. These items facilitate the identification of those elderly requiring specific services and interventions.

The Assessment of Living Skills and Resources (ALSAR) is an example of another instrument used to measure IADLs (Williams et al., 1991). This tool builds on earlier measures by incorporating the skill of the individual in completing each task as well as the resources available. It also combines the skill and resource scores to determine the ability of the individual to accomplish a task.

Skills and resources on the ALSAR are rated on scales of 0–2 with 0 being independent or adequate resources available. Functioning is assessed on 11 items associated with independent living. A risk score for each task is obtained. The total risk score for the items can be used in planning for services because it indicates specifically where more support is necessary.

As with the scales measuring the activities of daily living, important discrepancies exist among scales measuring IADLs. Scales may include as many as 16 activities that break larger functions into smaller tasks. Thus, dressing may be divided into activities such as combing hair, filing nails, and fastening buttons, while household chores may be subdivided into such distinct categories as turning a light switch on and off and turning a key in a lock (Kuriansky & Gurland, 1976). Scales may also include much more strenuous activities such as the ability to shovel snow, mow the lawn, or climb stairs. With these additions, more individuals may be categorized as disabled.

Differences in the wording of IADL instruments have significant consequences on the assessed status of older persons. As an example, a study using the OARS instrument on the noninstitutionalized elderly in Cleveland found them three times as functionally impaired as older persons in other parts of the United States. The wording of the IADL items on the OARS examines the ability to shop specifically for groceries and clothes. In comparison, the National Health Interview Survey inquires only about shopping for personal items. Using the more descrete measures in the OARS for assessment, the elderly in Cleveland are more likely to be defined as functionally impaired.

As with the ADL measures, there is no standardization regarding the categories of responses on the IADL instruments. Some record ability according to level of difficulty, ranging from "no difficulty" to "unable to perform with or without help." Others record the frequency of performing activities, while others rate each item on the degree of "problem" encountered in the performance.

Data on the ability to perform the IADLs is generally collected through self-reports or from the caregiver. Because of the complexity of the tasks, however, and the many factors that can influence performance, these assessments are not necessarily accurate. A critical limitation is that standardized instruments do not generally make allowances for the many variables that can influence both responses and abilities.

Ethnicity is one factor which can significantly affect the scores on IADL instruments. Depending on the degree of assimilation into American culture, many older ethnic or minority people may not be competent in IADL tasks. Those who are not fluent in English, who have remained within ethnic communities, and who have tended to rely on others to do shopping or manage their money are likely to score poorly on many measures, while actually functioning perfectly adequately within their traditional environments.

Gender, with its accompanying socialization differences, may also affect the scoring on IADL measures. Elderly men are frequently less competent in performing routine household chores, while older women may be less accustomed to decision making or managing finances. These factors, however, are frequently unaccounted for in measurements where one summary score records the amount of disability. Final scores may therefore not be reliable indicators of persons' actual ability to function.

A lack of motivation or a memory impairment on the part of the elderly person can severely affect both reported ability and/or performance. Depression, which can strongly influence mood may subsequently influence the validity of self-reported abilities. Thus, at any one time, the description of abilities may reflect more the current mental status of the individual than actual capacity for self-care. Moreover, measurements at any one time do not necessarily reflect usual performance ability.

Obtaining reports from family members does not necessarily improve those reports' validity; relatives are not necessarily knowledgeable about the individual's functioning. Moreover, the amount of impairment reported may reflect the amount of stress the caregiver experiences, rather than the actual status of the relative. Other motives, such as a desire to protect the older person or a desire to obtain more assistance can also influence these proxy responses.

COMBINED ADL AND IADL INSTRUMENTS

Instruments have sought to improve on the ADL/IADL scales by combining the measures as well as adding a measure of mental competence. The Hebrew Rehabilitation Center for Aged (HRCA) Vulnerability Index (Morris, Sherwood, & Mor, 1984) is composed of 11 items that can be completed through either self-report or by a proxy. Instrumental activities include meal preparation, taking out the garbage, and housework. ADLs consist of ability to walk up and down stairs, use of a walker or wheelchair, ability to dress self, and the number of days in a month that the individual went outside. In addition, it asks how much bad health or pain prevents the person from doing activities.

A combined ADL and IADL scale (Spector & Fleishman, 1998) uses 15 items that combine ADL and IADL measures. Respondents are asked whether they receive help from others on 7 ADL items, and if they are unable due to health to perform 9 IADL items. Analysis of the items shows no hierarchical relationship among them and that a simple sum of responses provides a measure of functional disability.

Most states use some measures of ADLs or IADLs in assessing eligibility to public service programs. A survey of criteria measures in 12 states reveals that all used the 6 traditional ADLs and the established set of 8 IADLs. However, states also expand these measures and may even assess social and environmental supports.

Findings from the survey show states also varying in the tasks used to determine dependency. For example, programs in Illinois inquire as to the ability to perform activities, the availability of assistance, and the frequency of its provision. The three scales are summed independently to provide a more sensitive measures of both functional need and service requirements.

The criteria for eligibility for community services varies even within states. Programs under the Older Americans Act (OAA), Medicaid waiver programs, and state-funded services as they vary in their targeting will also use distinct assessment measures. Under the OAA, services are intended to serve all persons over 60, but programs such as in-home services offered through Area Agencies on Aging may define their own eligibility criteria and target groups based upon local priorities and needs. However, given the emphasis placed on those with the greatest economic and social needs, services are charged with giving priority to elderly identified in those categories.

Under Medicaid waiver programs, most states provide services only to those low–income elderly who would otherwise be in a nursing home. Eligibility is therefore strictly defined according to precise ADL/ IADL measures.

State-funded programs usually have no income provisions and provide services based on functional limitations and client needs in conjunction with cost sharing. These assessments tend to rate the number of limitations in ADLs and IADLs, using the total score to estimate the need for service and what the client may have to pay. In many states, these scores are used in conjunction with the subjective assessment made by a case manager who has the final determination of eligibility.

Differences also exist with regard to the use of objective and subjective measures for assessing functioning. Systems may weigh and sum the scores across the individual functioning activities with eligibility decided by a specific numerical score. Others use this method in conjunction with the subjective evaluation of the person making the assessment, providing a more impressionable estimate of the degree of frailty and need.

Stone and Murtaugh's (1990) review of the implications of using differing criteria in the measurement of disability suggests how such criteria affect the elderly and the disposition of services. As an example, with a criterion of impairment in three or more ADLs lasting for at least 12 months, they estimate that there are 411,000 older persons eligible for home care services. If a less restricted criterion for eligibility is used, for example active or standby help required with any ADL or IADL lasting for at least 3 months, the estimate of those elderly eligible for home care increases to 4.1 million persons. Currently, under most federal programs, based on assistance needed in two or more ADLs, the number of eligible elderly is estimated at 857,000, but this could be expanded to 1.35 million if standby help is counted.

The usual criterion for eligibility for publicly sponsored services is a deficit in a minimum of two out of five ADLs: bathing, transferring, dressing, toileting, and eating. Those deficit in only one ADL are referred to as the moderately impaired and tend to be those able to function independently with the use of special equipment such as walkers or guard rails. It is important to also note that in using these criteria, the most common limitation found in community elderly is in bathing, while feeding and toileting show the least impairment.

The two-plus criteria is a commendable effort to assist in focusing services on those who are the most impaired in the community. However, using only the five core ADLs may exclude many who continue to have problems functioning due to mobility problems or difficulties in getting outside of the house. Many who could benefit from supports under the seven ADL assistance criteria are thus excluded from programs.

COGNITIVE IMPAIRMENT

In addition to physical impairments that limit functioning, frailty may result from cognitive impairment as it diminishes the capacity for independent living. Problems with memory, intellectual impairment, learning ability, calculation, problem solving, judgment, comprehension, recognition, orientation, and attention can severely impact on the ability to complete IADLs and may even affect the ADLs. Dementia, an illness whose prevalence increases with age, can particularly affect functioning capacity.

A recent survey of older persons in the community estimates that nearly one quarter of those over 65 have some cognitive impairment, with the proportion increasing by 10% every 10 years, with approximately one quarter developing dementia in 18 months (Unversagt et al., 2001). As dementia progresses, it results in declines in both the instrumental and basic activities of daily living (Schmeidler & Mohs, 1998).

Estimates of the extent to which these individuals require assistance with functioning is indicated in estimates from the Commonwealth Fund Commission. These indicate that over half of the 1.6 million severely impaired elderly persons living at home, those needing assistance with two or more ADLs are also cognitively impaired (Rowland, 1989). In fact, the likelihood of cognitive impairment rises with the number of ADL limitations. Whereas 22% of the elderly with two ADL impairments are cognitively impaired, the proportion increases to 44% of those with four or five ADL impairments.

As dementia can severely impede on functioning ability through behavior disorders and an inability to complete tasks required for living in the community, these individuals frequently require constant supervision, support, or direction in completing the tasks of daily living. However, impairments may not show up on traditional ADL/ IADL measures if questions are not worded to include the query, "Is supervision needed?" Without more precise measuring and wording of ADLs, assessments of functional ability in elderly with dementia are likely to be inaccurate (Hawes, 1990).

Measures of Cognitive Functioning

One of the most widely used instruments in the measuring of cognitive functioning is the Mini-Mental Status Examination (MMSE; Folstein, Folstein, & McHugh, 1975). The scale assesses orientation to time and place, recall, short-term memory, and ability to perform serial subtractions or reverse spellings.The test also measures constructional capacities by asking the person to copy a design, and the use of language by asking the subject to write a complete sentence. The results on each item are scored and summed together to provide a total maximum score of 30 points for the 11 items. A score of 23 points or fewer for a person with more than 8 years of education is evidence of cognitive impairment (Folstein, 1983). However, using the total score to judge the capacity for independent living may be an inaccurate assessment in that the individual may still be able to function adequately in his or her home environment.

The Brief Cognitive Rating Scale (BCRS; Reisberg & Ferris, 1983) measures the degree of cognitive impairment in concentration, recent memory, past memory, orientation, and functioning/self-care. The information is obtained from the subject, but in the presence of a caretaker, thus increasing the scale's validity. The advantage of this type of format is that completing the scale with the caretaker present can improve the validity of the responses, as denial often accompanies memory loss (Reisberg & Ferris, 1983). The instrument has seven categories for assessing self-care abilities ranging from "No difficulty"—either subjectively or objectively—to "Requires constant assistance in all activities of daily living."

Informant Measures

With regard to measuring actual ability to function in the community, other scales may be more relevant than the MMSE. The Dementia Rating Scale focuses on the ability to perform tasks associated with daily activities while also measuring memory and orientation. The information is provided by an informant who rates the subject's ability to cope with money, remember a three-item list, find his/her way indoors and around familiar streets, grasp explanations, and recall events within the last six months. The abilities to eat, dress, and toilet are scored separately.

The Blessed Dementia Scale (Blessed, Tomlinson, & Roth, 1968) is among the most widely used in gathering information from an informant. The ADL items include dressing, incontinence, and eating, while the IADL items include performing household tasks, managing money, finding the way indoors, familiarity with streets, interpreting surroundings, recalling recent events, ability to remember a short list, and tendency to dwell in the past.

The Cleveland ADL Scale (Patterson et al., 1992) includes 11 IADL items and 5 ADL items, dividing the ADL measures into subtasks that reflect initiation, appropriateness, and task completion. The use of subtasks such as selecting clothes, eating at appropriate times, and eating with acceptable manners increased the scale's sensitivity to ADL dysfunction.

The Bayer Activities of Daily Living Scale (B-ADL) focuses on assessing ADLs in persons in the community with mild to moderate dementia (Hindmarch, Lehfeld, deJongh, & Erzigkeit, 1998). The scale is comprised of 25 items and is completed by the caregiver or another person familiar with the patient. The B-ADL has been developed to be used internationally and reflect many domains essential to living at home.

The Functional Assessment Staging Scale (FASS; Reisberg, 1988) tracks changes through the course of Alzheimer's disease. The scale includes 16 items that measure IADLs, ADLs, and also role disability and communication impairment. The items are placed in order with the assumption that this order differs for demented and non-demented persons and that IADLs precede ADLs. The ADLs are ordered as dressing (choosing proper clothing), dressing (improper dressing without assistance or cuing), bathing, toileting, and incontinence. These items are followed by two communication items and by walking, sitting up, smiling, and holding up the head.

Performance Scales

Many instruments have been developed that measure performance of the person with dementia and are used to assess the ability for daily functioning. The Structured Assessment of Independent Living Skills (SAILS; Mahurin, DeBettignies, & Pirozzolo, 1991) measures a subset of ADLs (dressing and eating) and IADLs (telephoning, taking medications, and money management), as well as some motor tasks. Each subtask is scored from "unable" to "normal." There is also an item-specific intermediate level of disability as well as a judgment by the rater of the speed of the person in completing the task. The Direct Assessment of Functional Status (Lowenstein, Amigo, & Duara, 1989) focuses on IADLs and includes subtasks of telephoning, mailing a letter, managing money, and shopping. The items focus on memory, abstract reasoning, and orientation, and are scored as either correct or incorrect. Another scale, the Refined ADL Assessment (Tappan, 1994), measures five ADLs divided into subtasks with 5 to 21 physical steps per subtask. Functioning is assessed by responses which measure the extent to which verbal, visual, and physical prompts are needed for the subject to complete the specific tasks.

Limitations in Measures of Cognitive Impairment

An underlying issue with regard to defining the cognitively impaired as frail is that cognitive impairment does not necessarily correlate with functional dependency as measured by the ADLs. Many individuals who score poorly on mental status examinations may still be able to perform the ADLs without assistance. Thus, the inability to remember the date or to complete a sentence does not mean an inability to dress oneself or to bathe. On the basis of the ADLs alone, these individuals would not be identified as impaired, though they may be at risk of dependence with regard to the IADLs.

Another limitation with regard to the traditional instruments measuring cognitive capacity is that the items typically focus on attention, orientation, and memory, and ignore the capacity for decision-making. An elderly person might score reasonably high on the measures of recall and orientation but still be unable to make daily decisions essential for independent living. It is conceivable that one could accurately state the day and year but not be able dress, take medications, or remember the name of the physician.

A further issue in the measuring of cognitive functioning is whether the elderly person or the caregiver should be interviewed or provide the information. The two sources will not necessarily provide identical responses and it is not always easy to determine which is the more accurate. As with instruments measuring the ADLs, it is possible that the proxy respondent will either underestimate or overestimate the capacities of the subject. Obtaining information from both sources as well as using the subjective evaluation of the interviewer may be the optimal method for increasing validity.

In his discussion of instruments designed to measure functional disability in those with dementia, Spector (1997) finds that their validation is inconclusive but that they are correlated moderately with measures of cognitive impairment and generic measures of functional disability. There is also moderate correlation between performance measures and those of informants. At the same time, there is little consistency in the functional items included in the scales, with some predominantly ADL items and others focusing mainly on IADLs or combined items. In addition, it is not clear that informants actually understand the terms used in the measures.

MEASURES OF SOCIAL FUNCTIONING

Social functioning, the existence of social networks and the ability to interact with these important others who can provide emotional support as well as concrete assistance, are fundamental to the independence of many elderly. Impairments in social functioning imply that the older individual is restricted in interactions with others in the community who can play pivotal supportive roles essential for independence. Without such interactions and the ability to maintain these relationships, many elderly are at risk of forfeiting their independence.

Social functioning is a concept composed of many facets. Research shows that persons with strong social ties, social interactions, and emotional support are in better physical and mental health and better able to cope with ADL disabilities (Mendes de Leon, Gold, Glass, Kaplan, & George, 2001). In addition, having social contacts and participating in relationships may counteract disabilities, as these involvements motivate persons to continue to be engaged (Verbrugge, Reoma, & Gruber-Baldini, 1994; House, Landis, & Umberson, 1988).

On the other hand, receiving instrumental assistance with daily tasks has been found to increase disability risk (Mendes de Leon et al., 2001), suggesting that if persons become dependent upon others for assistance with daily tasks they may see themselves as increasingly disabled. Such dependency erodes the feelings of control or mastery that are important in assisting persons to adapt to functional declines and limitations (Mendes de Leon, Seeman, Baker, Richardon, & Tinetti, 1996). Consequently, caregivers are in a delicate position, as their emotional support can be critical to the adaptability of the older adult, while there is a risk that offering too much support that may erode feelings of self-efficacy.

With social functioning an important factor in the disability process, its measurement could be a critical part in determining needs for care. However, as the concept itself is diffuse, so are the scales used to define and assess it. Self-concept, self-esteem, life satisfaction, intergenerational relationships, social interactions, and the use of resources are all implied in the concept of social functioning. The extent to which each of these independently or together reflects functioning or needs is not clear.

A weakness in many instruments measuring social functioning is their failure to assess the respondent's satisfaction with the level of social involvement. This subjective evaluation is critical in that isolation or limited social relationships may be consistent with earlier patterns and not be indicative of poor functioning or predictive of frailty and support needs. Moreover, having infrequent visits with adult children does not imply that the elderly would not have their immediate support in case of illness or disability. This type of information is not uniformly reported on scales assessing social functioning, thus raising further questions about the validity of the measures.

As in the ADL and IADL instruments discussed earlier, there may also be discrepancies between responses given by the older individual and by an informant. Family members may want to underreport undesirable social behavior or overreport their own involvement, while the elderly subject may want to present a favorable impression to the interviewer and thus overreport family assistance and support. The validity and reliability of responses may therefore be seriously jeopardized.

The accuracy of measures of social functioning is questionable due to a lack of consistency in assessment, validity, and reliability. These weaknesses, as well as the continuing emphasis on physical ability as the main contributor to impairment, reinforce the neglect of social well-being in the assessment of frailty. Moreover, even when assessments of social functioning are made, they tend to not be given equal weight in determining service eligibility as either ADL or IADL measures.

Other areas significant to social functioning and the status of the older person are frequently not assessed. Measures of economic well-being remain difficult to assess or standardize because they vary among living situations, geographic areas, and even with the perceived needs of the respondent. The suitability and safety of the living environment, accessibility of services, and even the ability to drive a car are generally excluded from traditional measures. Thus, living in a high-crime area may severely restrict the autonomy of the older individual, while being unable to drive a car may force many others into isolation. In both instances, the affects of these environmental factors on functioning can be reductions in competency, social interactions, and the ability for self-care.

MULTIDIMENSIONAL ASSESSMENTS

Multidimensional assessment tools combine within one comprehensive instrument measures of several areas of functioning that are associated with general health, physical and mental functioning, and well-being. They typically measure behavioral competence, psychological well-being, environmental quality, and perceived quality of life. Because aging and disabilities involve many spheres of life as well as being interactive, these instruments can provide a more accurate description of the ability to function in the community.

The Older Americans Research and Service Center Instrument (OARS) is one of the oldest of the multidimensional instruments. It involves a 40–60-minute interview by a trained administrator who rates the subject on responses made on a 6-point scale in physical health, mental health, activities of daily living (both physical and instrumental), social well-being, and economic well-being. Scores are summed for each area and may be combined to represent an overall score representing the level of functioning.

The Multilevel Assessment Instrument (MAI; Lawton, Moss, Folcomer, et al., 1982) measures physical health, functional health, cognition, time use, social behavior, personal adjustment, and perceived environmental quality. It is administered by a trained evaluator, and like the OARS, provides scores in each area that can be combined into a composite index.

One of the most widely used instruments to measure health status is the MOS-36 (Ware & Sherbourne, 1992). It includes 36 items that measure limitations—in physical activities due to health; in social activities due to physical or emotional problems; in role activities due to physical health, bodily pain, and general mental health; in role activities due to emotional problems, vitality, and general health perceptions. As well as being performed by a trained administrator, it can also be self-administered or given over the telephone. It also has a single item that asks about health changes. The RAND-36 measure of health-related quality of life (Hays, Sherbourne, & Mazel, 1993) uses the same items but scores them differently. Both health-status scales have been widely used to assess health and quality of life although neither focuses particularly on older adults.

The use of comprehensive instruments has the advantage of showing a more valid measurement of the functioning of the older person, their supports, and their interactions. With the exception of health surveys and their occasional use by medical specialists, however, they are not routinely used as assessment tools. Programs and services that are responsible for providing for the care of older adults seldom use these more extensive measures. A lack of resources, including funds and trained staff and a lack of reimbursement procedures, are major obstacles to their utilization.

SUMMARY

Accurately determining needs for care is a complicated task requiring complex and comprehensive tools. Instruments for this process have been developed but are not routinely used. Most instruments continue to rely on measures of physical functioning which may be combined with measures of instrumental functioning. Weaknesses in both validity and reliability of these measures compromise their effectiveness. With so many instruments being used and each claiming to measure the same type of functioning, it is difficult to determine who is really at risk and in need of care.

Beyond the theoretical concerns associated with this limitation in measurement is the practical implication that it has on the lives of many elderly. Individuals in need of assistance are in danger of not receiving it because of the wording of a question or the absence of an item. It is conceivable that an individual could be judged frail and therefore eligible for services in one state, yet move to another state and be assessed as functionally competent and ineligible for support.

A weakness with many assessment instruments is their emphasis on objective criteria that fail to incorporate the subjective feelings of the older person. Objective criteria of measurement cannot assess the degree to which the individual feels vulnerable or at risk of dependency. Research has shown that even with chronic illnesses or problems in physical or cognitive functioning, a significant proportion of older adults will still rate themselves as aging successfully, while at the same time many elders without such conditions rate themselves as not aging successfully (Strawbridge, Wallhagen, & Cohen, 2002). These findings testify to the importance of obtaining subjective perspectives and ratings when attempting to determine and meet needs for care.

The measures used to assess eligibility for care are often a function of resources and the philosophy of those who control them. Moreover, the availability of resources may in itself affect the definition of functionality in that it may be more comprehensive and inclusive in periods of growth, while it becomes more exclusive in periods of recession, when resources are scarce. Using targeting as a measure to conserve resources can in itself have negative effects because it can neglect preventive and remedial services that could avert further the occurrence of dependency.

Policies and programs tend to target the most impaired, with few services available for those requiring only a small amount of assistance or supervision. In order to provide the support required for many elderly if they are to remain in the community, needs for care and dependency may best be viewed along a continuum. For many persons, providing care before functioning is severely impaired may prevent or delay further deterioration. The use of more comprehensive assessments is one factor that may help to ensure that this continuum is developed so that older persons receive appropriate care.

REFERENCES

Administration on Aging. (1965, amended). Older Americans Act. Hyattsville, MD: Author.

Blessed, G., Tomlinson, B., & Roth, M. (1968). The association between quantitative measures of dementia and of senile change in the cerebral gray matter of elderly subjects. *British Journal of Psychiatry, 114,* 797–811.

Brown, I., Renwick, R., & Raphael, D. (1995). Frailty: Constructing a common meaning, definition and conceptual framework. *International Journal of Rehabilitation, 18,* 93–102.

Coombs, S., Lambert, T., & Quirk, D. (1982). *An orientation to the Older Americans Act.* Washington, DC: National Association of State Units on Aging.

Duke University Center for the Study on Aging. (1978). *Multidimensional functional assessment: The OARS methodology* (2nd ed.). Durham: Duke University Press.

Fillenbaum, G. (1985). Screening the elderly: A brief instrumental activities of daily living measures. *Journal of the American Geriatrics Society, 33*(10), 698–706.

Folstein, M., Folstein, S., & McHugh, P. (1975). Mini-Mental State. A practical method for grading the cognitive state of patients for the clinician. *Journal of Psychiatric Research, 12*, 189–198.

Glass, T. (1998). Conjugating the tenses of function: Discordance among hypothetical, experimental, and enacted function in older adults. *Gerontologist, 38*, 101–112.

Gurland, B. J., Kurlansky, J., Sharpe, L., Simon, R., Stiller, P., & Berkett, P. (1977–1978). The comprehensive assessment and referral evaluation (CARE): Rationale, development and reliability. *International Journal of Aging and Human Development, 8*, 9–41.

Hawes, C. (1990). Selecting eligibility criteria for individuals with dementia. In M. Keean (Ed.), *Issues in the measurement of cognitive impairment for determining eligibility for long term care benefits.* Washington, DC: American Association of Retired Persons.

Hays, R., Sherbourne, C., & Mazel, R. (1993). The RAND-36-item health survey 1.0. *Health Economics, 2*, 217–227.

Hindmarch, I., Lehfeld, H., deJongh, P., & Erzigkeit, H. (1998). The Bayer Activities of Daily Living Scale (B-ADL). *Dementia, Geriatrics, and Cognitive Disorders, 9*, 20–26.

House, J., Landis, K., & Umberson, D. (1988). Social relationships and health. *Science, 241*, 540–545.

Jette, A. (1994). Physical disablement concepts for physical therapy research. *Physical Therapy, 79*(10), 939–948.

Kaethier, Y., Molnar, F., Mitchell, S., Soucie, P., Man-Son-Hing, M. (2003). Defining concepts of frailty: A survey of multi-disciplinary health professionals. *Geriatrics Today, 6*, 26–31.

Kovar, M., & Lawton, M. (1994). Functional disability: Activities and instrumental activities of daily living. *Annual Review of Gerontology and Geriatrics, 14*, 57–75.

Kuriansky, J., & Gurland, B. The performance test of activities of daily living. *International Journal of Aging and Human Development, 7*, 343–352.

Laditka, S., & Jenkins, C. (2001). Difficulty or dependency: Effects of measurement scales on disability prevalence among older Americans. *Journal of Health and Social Policy, 13*, 1–15.

Lawrence, R., & Jette, A. (1996). Disentangling the disablement process. *Journal of Gerontology, Social Sciences, 51B*, S173–S182.

Lawton, M., & Brody, E. (1969). Assessment of older people: Self-maintaining and instrumental activities of daily living. *Gerontologist, 9*(3), 179–186.

Lawton, M., Moss, M., Folcomer, M., & Kleban, M. (1982). A research and service oriented multilevel assessment instrument. *Journal of Gerontology, 37*, 91–99.

Liu, K., & Cornelius, E. (1989). *ADLs and eligibility for long term care services.* Report prepared for the Commonwealth Fund Commission on Elderly People Living Alone. Background Paper Series no. 14, Baltimore: The Commonwealth Commission.

Lowenstein, D., Amigo, E., & Duara, R. (1989). A new scale for the assessment of functional status in Alzheimer's disease and related disorders. *Journal of Gerontology, 44*, P114–P121.

Mahurin, R., DeBettignies, B., & Pirozzolo, F. (1991). Structured assessment of independent living skills: Preliminary report of a performance measure of functional abilities in dementia. *Journal of Gerontology, 46,* P58–P66.

Mendes de Leon, C., Gold, D., Glass, T., Kaplan, L., & George, L. (2001). Disability as a function of social networks and support in elderly African Americans and Whites: The Duke EPESE 1986–1992. *Journal of Gerontology, Social Sciences, 56B,* S179–S190.

Mendes de Leon, C., Seeman, T., Baker, D., Richardson, E., & Tinetti, M. (1996). Self-efficacy, physical decline, and change in functioning in community-living elders: A prospective study. *Journal of Gerontology, Social Sciences, 51B,* S183–S190.

Morris, J., Sherwood, S., & Mor, V. (1988). An assessment tool for use in identifying functionally vulnerable persons in the community. *Gerontology, 245*(4), 373–379.

Nagi, S. (1991). Disability concepts revisited: Implications for prevention. In A. Pope & R. Tarlov (Eds.), *Disability in America: A national agenda for prevention* (pp. 309–327). Washington, DC: National Academy Press.

Patterson, M., Mack, J., Neundorfer, M., Martin, R., Smyth, K., & Whitehouse, P. (1992). Assessment of functional ability in Alzheimer's disease: A review and a preliminary report on the Cleveland Scale for Activities of Daily Living. *Alzheimer's Disease and Associated Disorders, 6,* 145–163.

Pope, A., & Tarlov, A. (1991). *Disability in America: A national agenda for prevention.* Washington, DC: National Academy Press.

Powell, C. (1997). Frailty: Help or hindrance? *Journal of Research in Social Medicine, 90,* 23–36.

Reisberg, B. (1988). Functional assessment staging (FAST). *Psychopharmology Bulletin, 24,* 653–659.

Reisberg, B., & Ferris, S. (1983). A clinical rating scale for symptoms of psychosis in Alzheimer's disease. *Psychopharmacology Bulletin, 21,* 101–104.

Reuben, D., Valle, L., Hays, R., & Siu, A. (1995). Measuring physical function in community-dwelling older persons: A comparison of self-administered, interviewer-administered and performance based measures. *Journal of the American Geriatrics Society, 43,* 17–23.

Rowland, D. (1989). *Help at home: Long term care assistance for impaired elderly people.* The Commonwealth Commission on Elderly People Living Alone. Baltimore: The Commonwealth Fund Commission.

Schmeidler, J., & Mohs, R. (1998). Relationship of disease severity to decline in specific cognitive and functional measures in Alzheimer's disease. *Alzheimer's Disease and Related Disorders, 12,* 146–171.

Spector, W. (1997). Measuring functioning for the demented. *Alzheimer's Disease and Related Disorders, 11,* 81–90.

Spector, W., & Fleishman, J. (1998). Combining activities of daily living with instrumental activities in daily living to measure functional disability. *Journal of Gerontology B, Psychological Sciences and Social Sciences, 53,* S46–S57.

Stone, R., & Murtaugh, C. (1990). The elderly population with chronic functional disability: Implications for home care eligibility. *Gerontologist, 30,* 491–496.

Strawbridge, W., Shema, S., Balfour, J., Higby, H., & Kaplan, G., (1998). Antecedents of frailty over three decades in an older cohort. *Journal of Gerontology, 53B,* S9–S16.

Strawbridge, W., Wallhagen, M., & Cohen, R. (2002). Successful aging and well-being: Self-rated compared with Rowe and Kahn. *Gerontologist, 42,* 727–733.

Tappan, R. (1994). Development of the Refined ADL Assessment Scale for patients with Alzheimer's and related disorders. *Journal of Gerontological Nursing, 20,* 36–42.

Unversazgt, F., Gao, S., Baiyewu, O., Oguniyi, A., Gurege, O., Perskins, A., Emsley, C., Dickens, J., Evans, R., Musick, B., Hall, K., Hui, S., & Hendrie, H. (2001). Prevalence of cognitive impairment: Data from the Indianapolis study of health and aging. *Neurology, 57,* 1655–1662.

U.S. Department of Health, Education, and Welfare. (1978). *Public policy and the frail elderly.* DHEW Publication No. (OHDS) 79-20959. Washington, DC: Federal Council on Aging.

Verbrugge, L., Reoma, J., & Gruber-Baldini, A. (1994). Short-term dynamics of disability and well-being. *Journal of Health and Social Behavior, 35,* 97–117.

Ware, J., & Sherbourne, C. (1992). The MOS-36 item short-form health survey (SF-36). I. Concept framework and item selection. *Medical Care, 30,* 473–483.

Weiner, J., Hanley, R., Clark, R., & Van Nostrand, J. (1990). Measuring the activities of daily living: Comparisons across national surveys. *Journal of Gerontology, 45,* S229–S237.

Williams, J., Drinka, T., Greenberg, J., Ferrekk-Holton, J., Euhardy, R., & Schram, M. (1991). Development and testing of living skills and resources (ALSAR) in elderly community dwelling veterans. *Gerontologist, 31,* 84–92.

World Health Organization. (1980). International classification of impairments, disabilities, and handicaps. In *A manual of classification relating to the consequences of disease.* Geneva: Author.

Zimmerman, S., & Magaziner, J. (1994). Methodological issues in measuring the functional status of cognitively impaired nursing home residents: The use of proxies and performance based measures. *Alzheimer's Disease and Associated Disorders, 8,* S281–S290.

Chapter 3

Policy Affecting Care

Policy reflects the values and prevailing ideologies of society while also providing the framework for services. Responding to the community care needs of an aging society is a particularly pressing challenge to social policy, as it necessitates interventions at both the national and state levels. According to the Congressional Budget Office (CBO), national expenditures on nursing homes and community-based care will grow from $123 billion in 2000 to $346 billion in 2040, and this assumes a decline in the prevalence of functional disability (CBO, 1999). Such expenditures highlight the urgency of developing policies that offer humane and effective care.

The framework for such policies is generally subsumed under the rubric of long-term care. Although often confused with nursing home care, long-term care actually refers to a continuum of services providing an array of supports for the older or younger disabled person with reduced ability for self-care due to a chronic illness or impairment. In assessing needs for long-term care, measures of functional disability according to the activities of daily living and instrumental activities of daily living discussed in the previous chapter are often used.

Public financing through programs such as Medicare, Medicaid, the Veterans Administration, state programs, and the Administration on Aging fund the majority of both institutional and community-based services. Surprising to many older persons and their families is the fact that Medicare's coverage of long-term care, both nursing home and home care services, is restricted to eligibility criteria that stress a need for skilled services for a short period. Chronic illness that underlies most of the care needs of older adults is not covered.

Direct payments by families account for most of the private financing, approximately one quarter of the total costs of long-term care. Such costs can easily reach $4,500 or more per month (American Association of Homes and Services for the Aging, 2002). Private insurance, predominantly acute health care and Medicare HMOs, account for less than 7% of long-term care expenditures.

VALUES

With social values playing a key role in the development of policy, the issue of long-term care and who is responsible for it is under continual debate and scrutiny. One of the primary areas of debate is whether care is the responsibility of the individual, the family, or the government. Moreover, if it is a government concern, should it be under the purview of federal, state, or even local policy? Given these varying foci, it is little wonder that efforts to broaden and enhance long-term care to assure that it adequately addresses the growing needs of an aging society have been slow to develop or keep pace with changing needs.

This dilemma is intensified by traditional values that underscore the autonomy of the family and its independence from government in conjunction with values that stress individual responsibility. As these values tend to be shared by both policymakers and their constituents, it is not surprising that older adults needing assistance and their families face the burdens often associated with such care on their own, with little formal assistance or intervention. In fact, interventions are likely to be available and accessible only when the burden of care becomes overwhelming and informal resources are exhausted.

An inherent conflict exists between public support of dependent persons and the belief in self-reliance, autonomy, and protection from government intrusion. In a society that stresses productivity as a measure of self-worth, the actual value of those who are unproductive is sometimes questionable. At the same time, the belief in mutual support and the humanitarian ethic of providing for those less fortunate necessitates social responsibility for those unable to care for themselves.

Equity is a value that is implicit in American social policy, meaning that persons should be treated fairly and similarly in their receipt of benefits or services. At the same time, equity may be defined as being proportional—persons receive benefits in proportion to their need, or absolute—all receive equal benefits regardless of their level of need. Equity of access is particularly important in that it assures that all older persons in need of long-term care services have them regardless of age, gender, or income (Milbank Memorial Fund, 2000). However, equity in the provision of long-term care can be difficult to achieve if a primary policy concern is to reduce or control costs. In fact, the two aims, equity and cost containment, can be perceived as contending goals (Callahan & Wallach, 1981). Consequently, policymakers continue to struggle to balance the adequate provision of care to those in need with budget concerns.

Paternalism also pervades policies aimed at supporting older adults. This value is reflected in stereotypes and perceptions that view older persons with impairments as incapable of the same degree of self-fulfillment and self-realization as others in society. The result is that their options for self-determination can be severely limited as others are permitted to encroach upon their decision-making capacity and to act in their "best interest." As older persons with impairments are often unable to physically act on their decisions, they become vulnerable to coercion in long-term care (Collopy, 1988). Moreover, to the extent that persons are treated in a discriminatory way, they are at further risk of dependency and the loss of their individuality and rights.

Policymakers are cautious about infringing on individual rights, and at the same time, those in need may shun services that identify them as dependent or as not adequately fulfilling expected roles. Unfortunately, a reluctance to use formal services can further deter changes in policies because those in power may use such reluctance as evidence of an absence of need. With alterations in social policy made incrementally, any hesitation by potential service-users can further forestall changes that could make policies more comprehensive and relevant to meeting needs of impaired older adults.

Since the colonial period, the primary provider for the care of the elderly has been the family. Current policy continues to depend upon the family and is even built upon the premise that the family is and should be the primary party responsible for impaired older persons (Montgomery, 1999). Concurrently, there is concern that introducing formal services will reduce the family's involvement and increase dependency on the public system (Binney, Estes, & Humphries, 1993; Penning, 2002). However, data continue to underscore the major and dominant role of the family as care providers (National Long Term Care Survey, 1994). With major demographic changes, though, including more women in the workforce, intergenerational mobility, and increasing life span, the family is frequently unable to meet increasing care-giving responsibilities.

Evolving from traditions of the Elizabethan and Puritan societies, institutions have been the traditional places for care of dependent and impaired older persons without families or other informal supports. The poorhouses and almshouses of the colonial era became the nursing homes of American society, which have continued to act as the bulwark of care providers for those needing assistance. Consequently, community care, in order to obtain at least equal status as a provider, must continue to wrestle with this institutional bias.

Further reinforced by a medical framework that tends to treat dependency as a primary health condition, nursing homes, rather than the community, have been viewed as the most appropriate settings for the frail elderly. It is not surprising then, that in the year 2000, 72.5% of Medicaid dollars for long-term care was allocated to nursing homes, with just over one quarter, 27.5%, going to home- and community-based services (Special Committee on Aging, 2002).

GOALS

Policies are established to reach goals salient to society. The goal of a policy aimed at providing for the care of older adults in the community should be to assure that services are available and accessible to those in need. However, with a myriad of public and private programs involved in such care, each with its own distinct goals, it becomes difficult to discern one underlying policy goal. For instance, under Medicaid programs the primary goal is to meet the needs of those with limited financial means, while the goal of Medicare is to address acute medical needs that are temporarily limiting functioning but which that functioning can be restored.

If a policy goal is to provide support and assistance to older persons needing assistance to remain in the community, then the policy itself must be comprehensive with regard to who is entitled to services and what they may receive. The broader the definition of needs, the greater the number of persons that are entitled to services. Moreover, many factors, including social, mental, environmental, and cognitive impairments affect needs for assistance; an appropriate policy would encompass each of these areas. As an example, isolation or mild cognitive loss would be as important in determining eligibility as the ability to perform specific physical tasks.

One of the core dilemmas associated with policy goals for older adults is whether the policy is to be focused on prevention, maintenance, or restitution. Each of these implies a varying focus with appropriate practice strategies and interventions. Prevention encompasses health education, promotion, individual counseling, and even risk assessments. Maintenance involves supports and care that reduce or alleviate the risks of further deterioration, while restitution aims to enable the older person to regain some functions that had been limited.

Although the interventions associated with these goals are not necessarily exclusive, each is associated with specific activities that absorb scarce resources. Maximizing the older person's potential and supporting independence through community care are worthy policy goals, but require interventions in many areas in order to be reached. The diversity and fragmentation of policies and their goals often result in confusion with regard to service eligibility and benefits on the parts of both service providers and the intended consumers. Unfortunately, the older adults and their families to whom these policies and services are directed remain among the most vulnerable to this confusion.

EFFECTIVENESS

The fragmentation of policies complicates the development of any coherent system of services for meeting the needs of the older population, and makes it difficult to adequately assess their effectiveness. With goals remaining broad and undefined, it is difficult to determine the extent to which they are being reached or to evaluate the programs they mandate. In fact, this vagueness makes assessing the appropriateness of the goals themselves difficult. Effectiveness can only be measured when specific, well-defined objectives pertinent to the goals themselves have been developed. Given the plethora of policies dealing with the long-term care needs of older persons, such objectives are often difficult to identify.

POLICY AND INDIVIDUAL RIGHTS

The focus and intent of social policy is to provide solutions for major problems in society, solutions enacted or operationalized through various programs and services. Policies are not designed for individuals but for groups of people who share a common problem (Chambers, 2000). Focusing on the "greater good," however, may place many older persons at risk as the two guiding principles of our society, autonomy and self-determination, and the freedoms to make decisions and to act on them, may be overshadowed.

For the older adult in need of care, these freedoms revolve around interactions with both informal and formal supports that provide the assistance necessary for remaining in the community. The need for such assistance is in itself a threat to the continued independence and the ability to make decisions for the older person. This threat occurs because implicit in the interactions is the concept of "best interest," a term adopted from the medical profession. Beneficence directs the physician to promote and protect the best interests of the patient by seeking the greater balance of benefits over harm in treatment and care.

Within the broader framework of long-term care policy, best interest can enable others, family or agencies, to decide on services that they determine to be in the older person's best interests (Hofland, 1988). This dependence can, however, pose a threat to the individual's autonomy as the caregivers, both formal and informal, provide what they perceive is needed or is in the person's best interest—a perception that may or may not be congruent with the desires of the older person. The problem is most apparent when threats are posed to the person's independence due to concerns over his or her ability to function adequately in the community without assistance. Due to worry over the older person's welfare, family members and formal service providers may intervene and override the lifestyle or desires of the older adult. Though motivated by the best intentions, such interventions threaten autonomy and may even induce dependency.

Losing control over one's life increases the vulnerability to learned helplessness, a state characterized by diminished mastery over the environment (Maier & Seligman, 1976). Feelings of passivity and a tendency toward withdrawal associated with this state lead to decreases in self-esteem and well-being (Teitelman & Priddy, 1988). The nature of this learned helplessness can further impair an older person's interactions and coping abilities. Thus, the beneficence principle can accentuate the problem that it is attempting to resolve by creating further dependency.

GUARDIANSHIP

A fundamental issue in the provision of care to the impaired older adult is the process of providing assistance when the person is deemed incompetent to make decisions on his or her own behalf. Based on the doctrine of *parens patriae*, "father of his country," states are given the right and duty to protect those persons unable to care for themselves, as well as their property (Iris, 1988). This principle is enacted through the process of guardianship, by which individuals judged to be incompetent and unable to act on behalf of their own best interests are assigned legal guardians by the court. The use of guardianship in surrogate decision making has concomitantly increased with the growth of the older population (Bulcroft, Lielkoph, & Tripp, 1991). Risk factors for guardianship include increasing age, physical or emotional limitation small family networks, and not living with a spouse (Reynolds, 200⁵

A guardian is appointed by the court to make decisions for a person whom the court has judged to be incompetent in terms of self-care or money and estate management. Policy governing guardianship is designed and implemented at the state level, however, therefore many variations exist regarding its implementation.

There are two basic forms of guardianship. With "guardianship of the ward," the guardian is responsible for all aspects of the individual's life, and with "guardianship of the estate," he or she is responsible only for money and property. Underlying both is the assumption that the guardian will be acting in the "best interests" of the ward.

State laws specify the actions that guardians can take on their own and those that require prior court approval, with the courts approving fees for the guardian. Once granted, guardianship is seldom revoked. Guardianship can be requested by anyone, and in most states attorneys file a request with the probate court. The ward is entitled to legal representation at the hearing.

Other less restrictive alternatives to safeguarding the interests of the older person are "conservatorship" and "power of attorney." Conservatorship is a process whereby an individual asks the probate court to appoint a conservator to manage the property and finances of the older person. The court must find the person able to make the decision to have a conservator but unable to manage financial affairs. One of the few studies of conservatorship (Wilber, Reiser, & Harter, 2001) found that most persons were very impaired but that their estates were actually well managed. However, the conservatees reported feeling lonely and isolated, desiring more socialization and greater decision making in their own affairs.

Power of attorney gives the agent the power to make decisions, in spheres such as medical treatment, finance, or placement, on the ward's behalf. The person must be mentally competent in order to create a power of attorney. The power of attorney may be limited to only certain areas, such as health care or finances, or broad, covering all aspects of the person's life. It may also be non-durable, meaning that it takes effect immediately and usually for a specific transaction or until it is revoked. A durable power of attorney is continuous and will stay in effect if the person becomes incapacitated or mentally incompetent. A third type is a springing power of attorney, that only comes into effect when a person becomes incapacitated. Thus, it calls upon a third party to determine the capacity of the person to handle his or her affairs or make decisions, a judgment that may not always be congruent with a legal definition of competency.

Several issues with regard to guardianship, conservatorship, and power of attorney and safeguards to older adults can have enduring effects on their rights. Statutes regarding these legal roles vary among states, which adds to confusion for older persons and their families. In addition, there is no set method for determining competency, as states use varying tests to decide whether a person has the capacity to make decisions. Comprehensive medical assessments involving a history of the individual's previous behaviors, medications, or physical conditions that could influence a person's capacity are rarely required. At the same time, even with substandard evaluations, the vast majority of proceedings result in full guardianship (Dudley & Goins, 2003). To rectify this it has been suggested that three measures be used in measuring competency: a cognitive test, a behavioral test, and a test by the court that examines the individual's personal, environmental, and social context (Sabatino & Basinger, 2000).

Equally troubling is that power of attorney may be made without any competency assessment, so that an older person lacking judgment could be persuaded to give power of attorney to a person who could subsequently exploit him or her. In addition, there are few regulations regarding court-appointed attorneys acting as guardians. As monitoring of the work of these guardians is not routinely done, there is little control of their roles or performance, and much scope for abuse. There are few safeguards for the older person whose estate depends upon the integrity and ethics of this guardian.

A further concern regarding guardianship and the rights of the impaired older adult is that the evaluation of competency in one area does not necessarily coincide with other aspects of decision making. An individual may be unable to make a medical decision but be perfectly capable of functioning adequately at home. Full guardianship, rather than a limited guardianship restricted to only one aspect of decision-making, however, is often granted anyway.

Guardianship rests on the assumption that the appointed guardian will act in the interest of and according to the perceived wishes of the frail older person. The problem is that there are few guarantees to assure that these assumptions are upheld. Moreover, even with the best intentions, family members may not make decisions in accordance with the wishes of their relative. In some instances, their own emotional or financial situations may intervene in their treatment or care decisions. Basic to the protection of the interests of the older adult are the interactions within the family.

The "best interests model" incorporates the wishes and needs of bo' the older individual and the family in any decisions (Jecker, 1990). T model recognizes the interrelationship of the two units and is therefore sensitive to the interests and needs of each partner in decisions regarding future care. Although this model offers a sensitive means for assuring the perspectives and desires of both parties are recognized, there is little evidence that it is widely applied.

POLICY AND SERVICES

The government's involvement in the care of older adults is directly expressed through policies that mandate and offer support to specific programs and services. "Home- and community-based services" is the term often used to describe those programs whose goals are to enable persons with impairments to remain living independently as long as possible in the community, with a maximum sense of well-being.

Skinner (1990) classifies these programs into three basic categories: client assistance that provides income or benefits to support older persons; system optimizing that aims to ensure effective services; and service enhancement that directly funds providers to provide services to those in need. Although such programs may be offered in varying formats by the states, the federal policy offering the broadest foundation and support for these services is the Older Americans Act.

Older Americans Act

The enactment of the Older Americans Act in 1965 is the federal government's only comprehensive policy toward improving the lives of the older population. The original objectives included improving persons' lives in the areas of income, housing, employment, retirement, and community services, and assuring that older adults had freedom, independence, and the exercise of their own initiative in planning and managing their lives (National Association of State Units on Aging, 1982).

The act established the Administration on Aging as the institution in the federal government responsible for developing and offering services. Under Title III of the act, State Units of Aging were designated as the agencies responsible for developing and implementing state plans for services. Title III has remained the cornerstone of the act, as it is responsible for the array of supportive services that can enable persons to remain in the community.

Since the 1970s, amendments to the Older Americans Act have targeted services to the most vulnerable older persons, those with the greatest social and economic needs. These amendments recognize the importance of social factors including language barriers; cultural, social, or geographical isolation; ethnicity and race; as well as physical and mental impairment as factors that can restrict individual's ability to perform normal daily tasks and threaten their capacity to live independently. In the 1970s, amendments provided grants for funds for congregate meals and model projects to assist the physically and mentally impaired elderly.

The 1975 amendments mandated state and local agencies to develop programs in the areas of transportation and home services to assist the impaired elderly. System optimizing was to be accomplished through special funding allocated to ombudsman projects, services to meet the needs of those not being served adequately, and ambulatory day care services. These areas were consolidated in 1978 into three categories: access services (transportation, outreach, information, and referral); in-home services (home health aides, homemakers, telephone reassurance, chore maintenance); and legal services.

The 1987 amendments authorized funds specifically for non-medical in-home services for the frail elderly. This group includes those having a physical or mental disability, Alzheimer's disease or a related disorder with neurological or organic brain dysfunction that restricts the ability to perform daily tasks or to function independently. Amendments also required state plans to identify, coordinate planning for, and assess the service needs for older disabled individuals. The 1992 amendments placed greater focus on caregivers and added a new title, Title VII, Vulnerable Elder Rights Activities, that included the ombudsman program, prevention of elder abuse and neglect, elder rights and legal assistance, benefits outreach, and counseling.

The amendments of 2000 retained the focus on targeting low-income minorities and also added those living in rural areas. The emphasis on access services, in-home services, and legal assistance continues, with efforts to give more flexibility to states and area agencies on aging to develop their systems.

Particularly relevant to the care of the older adult in the community was the enactment in the 2000 amendments to the National Family Caregiver Support Program. The program provides funds to states to develop five basic services for family caregivers: information about services; assistance in gaining access to supportive services; individual counseling, support groups, and caregiver training; respite care; and supplemental services to complement the care given by caregivers. States may also allocate up to 10% of the caregiver funds for grandparents raising grandchildren. Priority is given to persons with the greatest social and economic need and to older adults caring for persons with mental retardation and developmental disabilities.

With its broad scope and focus on community and supportive services, and with the attention now being given to the informal caregivers of older adults, the Older Americans Act has the ability to truly address the many needs of older functionally impaired adults. However, its capacity to adequately meet these needs is challenged due to its limited funds. Funding for supportive services for the year 2000 was $325 million, with $125 million allocated for caregiver support services. Although funding has increased slightly each year, it has not kept pace with inflation and the growth of the older population (Kassner, 2001). Thus, it provides the foundation for services but has not been able to garner the appropriations essential for making them effective.

Americans with Disabilities Act/Olmstead Decision

Another policy that has the potential to address the care of the older adult in the community is the Olmstead Decision, made by the United States Supreme Court in 1999. The decision interpreted Title II of the Americans with Disabilities Act (ADA) by requiring states to administer services, programs, and activities to individuals with disabilities in the most integrated setting. It prohibits discrimination in public programs against persons with disabilities, and classifies as discriminatory any failure to make reasonable modifications in existing programs, although such changes are not required if it can be proven that they would alter the services. States are also asked to restructure existing programs to promote community integration and to establish individualized assessments for community placements. These may be reasonable assessments made by professionals to determine whether a person can safely live in the community.

The ADA gives positive impetus to developing services in the community for individuals with impairments, but the extent to which it will be fully implemented is difficult to determine. With shrinking budgets and fewer resources, states' abilities to develop such community programs will be compromised. Moreover, without a set time frame for changes, and with terms such as reasonable accommodation and reasonable assessments, programs will have a great deal of latitude in conforming to the act. Consequently, although the ADA underscores the importance of having all persons with functional impairments live in the least restrictive environment, its actual impact on the care of impaired older adults is uncertain.

Health Care

As older adults with impairments are primarily identified and defined according to physical disabilities that limit functioning, health care policy can be most relevant to addressing their needs. However, to a large extent, such policy fails in its role of meeting these needs as access to it remains limited, and for the most part, it fails to recognize the chronic health problems affecting functioning and independence.

Fundamental in the development of health care policy is the continuing debate on whether health care is a basic right to which all are entitled or a commodity to be purchased through private financing and expenditures. As a basic right, health care for all Americans would involve a universal and comprehensive program for which all with needs would be eligible and have equal access. When treated as a commodity, health care is something that is purchased, a condition placing it beyond the means of many. Many older adults, often those with the most impairments and the most vulnerable in the community, are unable to afford the health care services necessary to keep them independent.

Medicare

Medicare, Title XVIII of the Social Security Act, enacted in 1965, assists older persons with their health care expenditures. As a national insurance program for the elderly it offers universal coverage for the majority of Americans requiring hospitalization for acute medical problems. Under Medicare Part A, hospitalizations, limited stays in skilled nursing facilities, some home care, psychiatric hospitalizations, and hospice care are covered. Part B of Medicare covers payments to physicians, outpatient care, some mental health services, some preventive care, medical equipment, and some home health visits. As a government-sponsored program, it also attempts to curtail health care expenditures by reimbursing hospitals and physicians for reasonable costs only. Additionally, reimbursement for mental health care is half of that for other physician visits.

Medicare's applicability to the care of the functionally impaired elderly is limited in that it does not provide for chronic care. Coverage is severely limited for the types of services and items required by these older adults that can enable them to remain the community. Home care and day treatment services and reimbursements for items such as glasses, hearing aids, or dentures are restricted. Other equipment such as wheelchairs and lifts are subject to strict payment schedules and thus may be unavailable in regions of the country where Medicare coverage does not meet the fee charged by the supplier. Consequently, many older persons expecting to have their needs met through the Medicare program are shocked when they discover its restrictions and find that they lack expected supports that can assist them with their functioning.

Medicare underwent a significant programmatic change in 1983 when hospitals began to be reimbursed according to a patient's diagnosis. Hospitals were penalized by being refused reimbursement for days exceeding the specified period made in accordance with one of the more than 470 diagnostically related groups (DRGs) into which medical conditions are classified. Consequently, patients are at risk of being discharged either to a nursing home or to home before they are completely able to function. The impact on nursing homes is that they are often receiving very frail and sick persons who should have remained in hospital.

For those being discharged home, there is the concern that they will not be able to attend to all of their needs. The program operates under the assumption that once the acute condition is attended to, functioning will have been restored. But, as noted earlier, many older adults have multiple chronic conditions. Accordingly, their ability to care for themselves after discharge may be limited.

Home care services are geared toward those with acute conditions requiring skilled care. Although Medicare permits up to 35 hours of skilled home care services per week, limitations on payments to agencies through a prospective payment system make it unlikely that most persons will receive that amount of care. More importantly, the chronic health problems of older adults that affect functioning are generally not going to improve, and do not qualify for skilled home care. Consequently, Medicare's role in providing for these problems remains limited.

The Balanced Budget Act of 1997 created the Medicare+Choice program to enable beneficiaries to enroll in and take advantage of managed care organizations. The program was perceived as a way to lower and contain health care costs while enabling participants to obtain additional benefits such as prescription drugs, vision care, and preventive dental care. Many plans did not charge enrollees more than their Part B premium from Medicare, with providers paid a fixed amount per member per month. In the last few years many plans have restricted accepting high risk older patients who would generate higher costs. At the end of 2002, nearly 217,000 Medicare beneficiaries were dropped by their HMOs as plans withdrew from the Medicare+Choice program (Barry, 2002), raising doubt regarding the extent to which these plans can meet the needs of the chronically ill older population.

The impaired older patient with complex medical conditions presents a challenge to physicians in terms of both their time and skill (Butler & Hyer, 1989). The comprehensive geriatric assessment particularly pertinent to the needs of these patients and to the development of an appropriate care plan are not reimbursed under Medicare. Care coordination, counseling, and education that can also be critical in meeting the many needs of the patient are demanding tasks, often requiring the involvement of several professionals, but are areas that are not covered under present Medicare reimbursement.

In recognition of these needs, the Geriatric Care Act of 2003 was introduced in Congress in an effort to expand medical residency training in geriatric medicine and offer reimbursement for care coordination and assessment services under Medicare. If enacted, the bill would permit initial and annual assessments of medical conditions, functional and cognitive capacity, and environmental and psychological needs, and would be a definite recognition of the needs of these patients.

The geriatric care bill also calls for the coordination of medical and other health services for those with serious and disabling chronic conditions, and patient and family education and counseling. These services would be provided to those with ADL restrictions or those requiring supervision due to cognitive impairments that act as threats to their health and safety.

After years of debate and many proposals, Congress passed a prescription drug package under Medicare in 2003. The new legislation goes into effect in 2006, and includes a higher monthly premium and involves some cost-sharing, while offering greater financial assistance to those below the poverty line than to middle- or higher-income older persons.

For the first time, Medicare will impose a means test on participants, with persons earning more than $80,000 per year paying a higher premium for physician visits and outpatient services. Private health insurance plans will receive subsidies to encourage them to cover older persons and the disabled. The legislation further underscores the continued importance of the Medicare program and the urgency of further developing the program so that it can meet the needs of the older population.

Medicaid

Medicaid, Title XIX of the Social Security Act, created in 1965, is a joint federal and state assistance program for the poor and medically indigent. The federal match to state dollars ranges between 50% and 77% based on state per-capita income. Since its inception, it has become the largest single public payor of health and related services for chronically impaired older adults. In 2000, Medicaid covered 45% of long-term care costs in the country, in comparison with 14% covered by Medicare. Although the elderly account for only one quarter of the enrollees, they account for two thirds of the spending, with Medicaid covering 50% of all nursing home costs (Kaiser Family Foundation, 2002). The majority of Medicaid expenditures are made to nursing homes, with a much smaller proportion going to home- and community-based care.

States administer their own programs, determining, within federal guidelines, eligibility and benefits. For those requiring long-term care services, the federal government requires that nursing home care and home health care are offered. The home health care benefit covers nursing, home health aides, medical supplies and equipment, and physical and other therapies.

Under the Personal Care program and the Home and Community Based Care Waiver Program (HCBC), states can provide increased benefits in the home to persons who would otherwise be institutionalized. These benefits include homemaking, case management services, respite care, and adult health as well as other services. States vary considerably with regard to services provided under the waiver program and in the services that they offer. Under the waiver states have been able to develop demonstration programs for new types of health care delivery, including managed care.

Since the 1990s, however, state budgets have been considerably reduced, while unemployment rates have risen along with the numbers seeking Medicaid assistance. Increases in medical costs as well as the costs associated with long-term care have begun to impact Medicaid programs. A study of states offering waiver services in 1997 found most states reporting that they had inadequate slots for clients and waiting lists for program services (Harrington, LeBlanc, Wood, Satten, & Tanner, 2002). The survey found that barriers to expanding HCBS include inadequate numbers of suppliers, limited state legislative support for the programs, and federal regulatory barriers such as restrictions on need criteria.

Many states are taking measures to reduce Medicaid expenditures by controlling the costs of prescription drugs, increasing eligibility requirements, decreasing benefits, and reducing home health care (Kaiser Family Foundation, 2002). All of these constrictions could have major ramifications on the scope of the services offered to older adults.

In an effort to relieve the financial burden that nursing homes can place on federal and state funds, the Medicaid State Recovery for Long Term Care provisions were enacted in 1993 as part of the Omnibus Reconciliation Act. This legislation requires states to recover the costs of nursing home and other long-term care services from the estates of beneficiaries with states required, at a minimum, to file claims in probate court against certain estates. There is little data on the impact of this recovery with regard to state budgets, and it is not clear how the threat of such actions may affect persons' willingness to enter the Medicaid program.

Title XX and the Omnibus Budget Reconciliation Act

Other major federal policies with an impact on the frail elderly are Title XX of the Social Security Act and the Omnibus Budget Reconciliation Act. Title XX, passed in 1974, designated the federal government to allocate funds to the states for supportive social services for low-income persons. The objectives of these services were to increase self-sufficiency, deinstitutionalization, and home-based care. Although the elderly were not directly identified as a targeted group, the goals of the act addressed their needs by virtue of income status and the programs offered. Title XX is a major provider of services such as home-delivered and congregate meals to elderly recipients of Supplemental Security Income.

The Omnibus Budget Reconciliation Act of 1981 (OBRA) amended Title XX by creating a Social Services Block Grant (SSBG), to be given to states with funding based on a formula according to the size of their populations. The SSBG transferred authority for services to the states while also reducing federal spending. States were given the power to decide on what programs to offer and eligibility criteria. OBRA broadened the scope of Title XX by rescinding the requirement that 50% of the recipients had to be participants in Medicaid, Supplementary Security Income, or Aid to Dependent Children programs.

The types of services most frequently provided to low- and moderate-income older persons are for community services such as homemakers, chore services, home health, adult protective services, adult day care, transportation, and nutrition programs. The grants also fund adult protective services to prevent abuse, neglect, and exploitation.

It is important to note, however, that only a small proportion of the funding goes to the older population. Moreover, SSBG funding has been cut by over $1 billion in the last several years. Although states are allowed to transfer a small percentage of their Temporary Assistance to Needy Families (TANF) funds to the SSBG, such transfers can be made only to programs serving families and children; transfers cannot be made to programs for the vulnerable elderly. With funding continuing to be limited, the viability of SSBG's role in supporting community care services for older persons is in jeopardy.

POLICY FOR FAMILY SUPPORT

In 1997, one in four United States households (22.4 million) was involved in family caregiving for an older relative (National Alliance for Caregiving & American Association of Retired Persons, 1997). Data from the survey indicated that the average family caregiver devotes 18 hours per week to caregiving tasks, with 18% of caregivers giving 40 hours of care per week. As well as providing the bulk of long-term care services, these caregivers, by maintaining their relatives in the community, often through their own funds, provide vast cost savings for the government. Federal support for these caregivers is limited, although many states have developed their own innovative and unique programs to assist them.

The United States remains one of the few industrialized countries without a national policy in support of family caregivers. Federal family allowances, stipends, and payments to caregivers common in European countries have yet to be enacted here. A primary source of assistance in the United States is the child and dependent care credit. This permits a working caregiver to deduct expenses paid to a nonrelative caregiver caring for a dependent spouse or another person who is physically or mentally unable to care for himself/herself. The expenses for this dependent care is available for the person while looking for work as well as during employment. Caregivers are able to deduct a percentage of those expenses, up to a scheduled maximum amount, from their federal income tax.

As a measure of financial support for caregivers, the tax credit provides only limited assistance. Moreover, for nonworking caregivers, the credit has little relevance. Consequently, the majority of caregivers do not receive any federal subsidies. Those receiving the most benefit from the credit are those with lower incomes, since the proportion of tax credits they receive is higher than for those with greater incomes. Even these credits, though, may not realistically approach the actual costs of care.

The National Family Support Act funded through the Administration on Aging discussed earlier in this chapter was allocated $155 million in FY 2003 with a decrease proposed by the administration to $142 million in FY 2004. The legislation directs the Area Agencies on Aging to use their allotted funds to provide caregivers with information, access to services, counseling, support groups, and caregiver training, respite care, and supplemental services. Given the vast number of caregivers and their many needs, the potential for the legislation to have a real impact without more substantial funding must be questioned. However, the program is important in that it does give formal recognition to caregivers at the federal level.

The Federal Family Leave Act is further formal recognition of the needs that families have in relation to caregiving and that these needs are not restricted to childrearing. The act permits an employee to take up to 12 weeks of unpaid leave per year to provide care to a seriously ill parent or spouse. However, the act pertains only to employers of 50 or more persons. Employees' benefits must be maintained during the leave period and their jobs must be restored on their return.

Further progress with regard to family caregivers is reflected in the number of bills that have been introduced in Congress in the last few years. Bills to assist families in obtaining respite, that would give income tax credit to caregivers caring for a relative with long-term care needs, and one that would help caregivers accumulate Social Security credits when taking time off from work for caregiving. Through the attention and advocacy such legislation generates, these are major steps in further recognizing the roles and needs of family caregivers.

PRIVATE SECTOR POLICIES

A major focus in the private sector with regard to care is long-term care insurance. The interest in long-term care insurance began in the 1980s, with the idea of a policy that persons could purchase to help protect their assets and cover the expenses of long-term care services. In 1990, fewer than 2 million policies had been sold, but by the year 2000 this number had increased to more than 6 million (Health Insurance Association of America, 2000). However, these policies pay less than 10% of the country's total expenditures on long-term care (Congressional

Record Services, 2000). Most policies are sold to individuals, although increasing numbers of employers, as well as the federal government, provide policies to their employees.

The policies typically reimburse the costs of nursing home care, assisted living, home care, adult day care, and other chronic care services. Given the continued rise in the costs of services, however, it is critical that the policies give inflation protection. Research suggests that a 5% compound inflation rider should be adequate for most policyholders, though this also depends upon a continued shift from nursing home to community- and home-based care (Cohen, Weinrobe, & Miller, 2002). Even with this rider, nursing home costs may exceed the policy benefit, while those remaining in the community may find themselves overinsured.

The cost of long-term care insurance remains high and therefore beyond the reach of persons with limited resources. Policy costs increase with age and thus as many persons reach the age when they begin to consider purchasing a policy, it is at a time when the premiums may be most expensive. For younger persons raising families, immediate concerns about inflation and resources can act as deterrents to purchasing the insurance. Attitudes regarding family responsibility, the role of government, and a lack of information about the risk, current coverages, and the availability of the insurance can also act as deterrents (Weinick, Weigers, & Cohen, 1998). Policies offered by employers are the most likely to be purchased.

CONSUMER-DIRECTED SERVICES

Many states have developed consumer-directed personal care programs in which older persons assess their own needs; determine by whom and how these needs should be met; and remain responsible for monitoring the help that they receive. The intent of consumer direction is to permit the consumers themselves to assess their own needs and determine how they should be met, as well as monitor the care they receive. Consumer direction can range from giving individuals complete independence in making decisions and arranging services, to having fiscal intermediaries assist in managing services.

Cash and counseling demonstration programs were implemented in 1996 in four states, to assess the approach of giving Medicaid recipients the choice of receiving traditional services from agencies or cash with counseling assistance. The counseling assists them with information and assistance in choosing and arranging services, and assuring that the funds are spent appropriately. The cash may be used to purchase services from a traditional home care agency, to pay a friend or relative for providing care, to make home modifications, or to arrange for other personal assistance. The intention of all of these services is to assist persons to continue to live independently in the community.

Supportive of the interest by older persons in this type of program are findings from a national survey of persons 50 years and older, which found that almost half, 46%, wanted more direct control over the services they receive. It is interesting to note that ethnicity may impact this preference, as another study comparing the interests of African American, Chinese, Latino, and White older consumers found that overall, 73% favored a traditional case-management model, with the care managers making decisions and arranging for care (Sciegaj, 2001).

A review of programs in four states (Coleman, 2003) shows a high level of satisfaction among older participants, with most persons believing that the quality of their lives has improved by directing their own services. In many instances service satisfaction appears to be related to being allowed to hire family members. However, the review also indicates that older consumers differ in the extent of control they want over the services and the workers. Among the recommendations given are that states should provide options so that a range of control is possible: backup services should be available, persons should be permitted to return to traditional programs if management on their own is no longer possible or desired, and consumer direction should be voluntary.

The largest consumer-directed program in the country is that of California. This state requires that the program is offered in all counties to persons eligible for Medicaid. Assessments are made of the participant's functional and cognitive status to determine the needed number of monthly hours of services, with the maximum being 238 hours. Personal care, assistance with household chores, paramedical supervision, protective supervision, and medical transportation are among the provided services.

The consumers are responsible for recruiting, hiring, training, and supervising the workers, who may be family members. Monthly budgets are calculated on the number of service hours multiplied by the hourly wage of the worker which varies with the county. In 2003 hourly wages ranged from $6.75 to $10.50, with the average monthly payment for services approximately $698.00.

Research on the outcomes of the program (Doty, Benjamin, Matthia, & Franks, 1999) found that slightly more than half of the participants over the age of 65 hired family members as their care providers. In comparison to persons using a professional agency model rather than consumer-directed care, those in the consumer-directed program had less worker turnover in a year but reported more problems finding a backup worker in case of an emergency. Both groups were generally satisfied with their care; however, the consumer-directed participants reported greater compatibility with their workers.

Consumer-directed care is an empowering rather than debilitating approach to providing assistance to older adults. As it builds upon their strengths it fosters their capacity for autonomy and decision making, and has the potential of increasing their ability for independence. At the same time, such programs can be particularly cost effective for states by helping to maintain persons in the community and reducing the administrative costs associated with the provision of agency services. Consequently, such programs may play major roles in the future development of long-term care.

SUMMARY

Policy is essential for the development of services to address needs of older persons in the community. Policies reflect a society's ideologies and values and consequently are major influences on the ways in which services are defined and offered. In the United States, policy toward the care of older persons requiring assistance continues to wrestle with the roles of the individual and the family vis-á-vis those of the government and public support. Community care continues to compete with a tradition that has favored institutions as the primary sites for the care of dependent elderly. This tradition is reinforced by a perspective that perceives impairments primarily as medical problems to be treated by the health care system.

In order to best meet the needs of older persons in the community, policies must be comprehensive and able to address the many areas of a person's life that may affect their functioning and ability to remain independent. To the extent that policies remain fragmented, their effectiveness is severely compromised. In addition, care must be taken that the rights of the individual are recognized and that impairment in one area is not used to assume that the person is unable to make decisions regarding their own lives or care. Consumer-directed programs offering older persons the ability to decide on and govern their own care and services are important mechanisms for fostering independence and autonomy.

The Older Americans Act (OAA) provides the foundation for most community care services in this country. Throughout the years, this act has continued to target the needs of the most vulnerable in the community by aiming to provide services that help to support them. Most recently, the OAA has further recognized the importance of the family as care providers by designating funds specifically for family caregivers. However, the effectiveness of the act itself in meeting its goals remains restricted, due to the failure of funding levels to meet the demand for services. Funding also affects the effectiveness of other federal programs such as the Americans with Disabilities Act and the Omnibus Reconciliation Act of 1987. Each offers the foundation for services but lacks the resources to support them.

The role of Medicare in meeting the needs of older persons in the community remains limited, as it continues to focus on acute rather than chronic care needs that can impact functioning. The role of Medicaid in providing community care is also limited in that the majority of its expenditures continue to be for institutional rather than home and community services. Through its waiver program, states are able to offer a large array of services that can assist persons to remain in the community, but the provision of these services depends to a large extent on state budgets.

The United States remains one of the few developed countries without any national policy in support of the family. Although some legislation has been passed that acknowledges the needs of family caregivers, it is questionable that it can truly influence the well-being of families and their ability to continue to provide care. At the same time, the recognition of their roles in caring for older persons offers the basis for further policy initiatives.

A true commitment to community care requires recognizing the home and community as the most appropriate environments for meeting care needs of older persons. This commitment necessitates a comprehensive policy that takes into consideration the ways in which the needs of older persons are interrelated and affected by a myriad of factors. Policy to serve older persons in the community is as complex as the needs of the population itself, but as long as it remains fragmented, it will be limited in effectively addressing these needs. Viable community care requires a comprehensive focus and a policy that assures that services are widely available and not dependent upon an individual's personal resources.

REFERENCES

American Association of Homes and Services for the Aging. (2002). *Broken and unsustainable: The cost crisis of long-term care for baby boomers.* Washington, DC: Author.

Barry, P. (2002). More HMOs Leave Medicare. *AARP Bulletin, 43,* 10. Public Policy Institute, AARP, Washington, DC.

Binney, E., Estes, C., & Humphries, S. (1993). Informalization and community care. In C. Estes, J. Swan, & Associates (Eds.), *The long-term care crisis: Elders trapped in the no-care zone* (pp. 155–170). Newbury Park, CA: Sage.

Bulcroft, K., Lielkoph, M., & Tripp, K. (1991). Elderly wards and their legal guardians: Analysis of county probate records in Ohio and Washington. *Gerontologist, 31,* 156–165.

Butler, R., & Hyer, K. (1989). Reimbursement reform for the frail elderly. *Journal of the American Geriatric Society, 37,* 1097–1098.

Callahan, D., & Wallach, S. (1981). *Reforming the long term care system.* Lexington, VA: D. C. Heath & Co.

Chambers, D. (2000). *Social policy and social programs* (3rd ed.). Boston: Allyn & Bacon.

Cohen, M., Weinrobe, M., & Miller, J. (2002). *Inflation protection and long-term care insurance: Finding the gold standard of adequacy.* Washington, DC: Public Policy Institute, AARP.

Coleman, B. (2003). *Consumer-directed home services for older people in the U.S.* Washington, DC: Public Policy Institute, AARP.

Collopy, B. (1988). Autonomy in long-term care: Some crucial distinctions. *Gerontologist, 28,* 10–18.

Congressional Budget Office. (1999). *CBO memorandum; projections of expenditures for long-term care services for the elderly.* Washington, DC: Author.

Congressional Record Service. (2000). *Long-term care chart book: Persons served, payors, and spending.* Washington, DC: Author.

Doty, P., Benjamin, A., Matthia, R., & Franks, T. (1999). *In-home support services for the elderly and disabled: A comparison of client-directed and professional management models of service delivery.* Washington, DC: U.S. Department of Health and Human Services, Office of the Assistant Secretary for Planning and Evaluation.

Dudley, K., & Goins, R. (2003). Guardianship capacity evaluations of older adults: Comparing current practice to legal standards in two states. *Journal of Aging and Social Policy, 15,* 97–115.

Harrington, C., LeBlanc, A., Wood, J., Satten, N., & Tanner, C. (2002). Met and unmet need for Medicaid home and community-based services in the states. *Journal of Applied Gerontology, 21,* 484–510.

Health Insurance Association of America (HIAA). (2000). *Who buys long term care insurance in 2000: A decade of study of buyers and non-buyers.* Washington, DC: Author.

Hofland, B. (1988). Autonomy in long term care: Background issues and a programmatic response. *Gerontologist, 28,* 3–10.

Home and Community Based Services. (2001). *States moving forward on Olmstead planning.* Downloaded April 1, 2004 from http://www.hcbs.org/new/ncsl_olmstead_study.htm

Hospital and Healthcare Compensation Service. (2000). *Home care salary and benefits report, 2000–2001.* Oakland, NJ: Author.

Institute of Medicine. (2000). *Improving the quality of long term care.* Washington, DC: National Academy Press.

Iris, M. (1988). Guardianship and the elderly: A multiperspective view of the decision-making process. *Gerontologist, 28,* 39–45.

Jecker, N. (1990). The role of intimate others in medical decision making. *Gerontologist, 30*(1), 65–71.

Kaiser Family Foundation. (2002). *Medicaid spending growth: Results from a 2002 survey.* Washington, DC: Author, Kaiser Commission on Medicaid and the Uninsured.

Kassner, E. (2001). *The role of the Older Americans Act in providing long term care.* Washington, DC: Public Policy Institute, American Association of Retired Persons.

Maier, S., & Seligman, M. (1976). Learned helplessness: Theory and evidence. *Journal of Experimental Psychology: General, 105,* 3–46.

Milbank Memorial Fund & World Health Organization. (2000). *Towards an international consensus on policy for long-term care of the aging.* New York: Milbank Memorial Fund.

Montgomery, R. (1999). The family role in the context of long term care. *Journal of Aging and Health, 11,* 383–416.

National Alliance for Caregiving & American Association of Retired Persons. (1997). *Family caregiving in the U.S.: Findings from a national survey.* Bethesda, MD: AAC/AARP.

National Association of State Units on Aging. (1982). *An orientation to the Older Americans Act.* Washington, DC: Author.

National Institute on Aging & Duke University Center for Demographic Studies. (1994). *National long term care survey.* Arlington, VA: National Institutes of Health.

Penning, M. (2002). Hydra revisited: Substituting formal for self- and informal in-home care among older adults with disabilities. *Gerontologist, 42,* 4–16.

Reynolds, S. (2002). Guardianship primavera: A first look at factors associated with having a legal guardianship using a nationally representative sample. *Aging and Mental Health, 6,* 109–120.

Sabatino, C., & Basinger, S. (2000). Competency: Reforming our legal fictions. *Journal of Mental Health and Aging, 6,* 119–143.

Sciegaj, M. (2002). *Elder preferences for consumer-directed community care: Implications for policy and management.* Waldham, MA: Brandeis University, Schneider Institute for Health Policy.

Skinner, J. (1990). Federal programs for the vulnerable aged. In Z. Hazel, P. Ehrlich, & R. Hubbard (Eds.), *The vulnerable aged: People, services and policies.* New York: Springer Publishing.

Special Committee on Aging, U.S. Senate. (2002). *Long term care report.* Washington, DC: U.S. Government Printing Office.

Teitelman, J. L., & Priddy, J. M. (1988). From psychological theory to practice: Improving frail elders' quality of life through control-enhancing interventions. *Journal of Applied Gerontology, 7*(3), 298–315.

Weigers, M., Weinick, R., & Cohen, J. (1998). Children's health insurance, access to care, and health status: New findings. *Health Affairs, 17*(2), 127–136.

Wilber, K., Reiser, T., & Harter, K. (2001). New perspectives on conservatorship: The views of older adult conservatees and their conservators. *Aging: Neuropsychology, and Cognition, 8,* 225–240.

Community Programs and Services

Programs and services are designed to meet the specific goals of a policy. The extent to which they are able to do so is largely determined by the amount of resources allocated to the programs, as well as by the ways services are delivered. Ideally, community programs for impaired older adults should seek to foster autonomy, recognize the self-determination and desires of the individual, and offer options with regard to service.

In designing community programs for older adults, varying schemas have been developed. The Gerontological Society of America (1978) categorizes services based upon the degree of impairment of the intended population group: unimpaired, minimally impaired, moderately impaired, and severely impaired. Using this type of classification, services can be offered in terms of the status of the group: preventive for the unimpaired; supportive for the moderately impaired; protective for the severely impaired. Depending on the level of needed services, decisions can also be made as to whether care is best provided in the community or in an institution (Monk, 1990).

Other classification schemes group services according to whether they are primarily client assisting, service enhancing, or system optimizing (Skinner, 1990). An example of a client assistance service is one that offers financial support or other types of benefits. System optimizing services aim to increase the effective use of programs by monitoring the rights of the intended consumers to assure that they are receiving appropriate care. Service enhancement programs fund service providers so that they may continue to develop services according to the needs of the older impaired population.

Programs have also been grouped according to whether they are community-based, home-based, congregate-residential, or institution-based. Each group can serve varying levels of functionally impaired persons, indicating that many impaired persons can be cared for in the community in less restrictive settings than in institutions (Tobin & Toseland, 1990).

The problems involved in the classifying of services are reflected in the programs funded under Title III of the Older Americans Act, the title responsible for authorizing and funding home- and community-based services. Under Part B of the act, Area Agencies on Aging (AAAs) receiving funding must provide assurances that adequate funds will be provided for access, in-home and supportive services, senior centers, and legal services. Access includes case management, transportation, information and referral, and outreach. In-home services include home-maker, chore, and supportive services for caregivers of persons with Alzheimer's disease and other dementias. Supportive services include health and mental health care, transportation, information and assistance, housing, long-term care, supportive activities for caregivers, in-home services for the frail, legal assistance, programs that encourage employment of older workers, and crime prevention.

Title III C-1 provides funds for congregate meals and home–delivered meals. Part D funds programs in disease prevention and health promotion and Part E is the national Family Caregiver Support Program, which includes assistance to family caregivers, information, counseling, respite care, and supplemental services that can complement care.

However, much overlap remains between categories and services. This overlap can affect the ways in which AAAs and states report their data, according to their own needs and criteria for classifying services and the various populations served. Transportation services and caregiver support programs could be classified and funded under at least two programs. Although this gives states greater flexibility in the use of funds, it also makes it more difficult to determine gaps in services and further needs for expansion at a national level. Consequently, confusion over how to report or classify service utilization can impact program planning and determining resource needs. At the same time, the blurring of boundaries reflects the reality of needs of older persons requiring assistance. For example, day care supports both the individual and the family, while transportation is critical for both access and support.

A major concern underlies service utilization: Even though different levels of impairment may relate to a need for varying levels of services, all services are not necessarily available in every community. In addition, inadequate funds and program resources mean that in many areas needs cannot be met.

SERVICE UTILIZATION

Although services may be available to assist older adults who have disabling conditions and functional limitations, availability does not imply actual use. Reaching persons in need of assistance and engaging them in the service network, particularly those most in need, remains a challenge.

Studies of service utilization have relied heavily on the model of health service utilization developed by Anderson and Newman (1973). The model perceives service use as being predicted by three groups of factors: predisposing, enabling, and need. Predisposing factors include sociodemographic characteristics, attitudes, and previous experiences. Enabling factors can include transportation, income, insurance, and informal supports, and need is the individual's perceived need for the service and conviction that it will help. A review of research regarding the importance of these factors in predicting service use found those associated with perceived need to be the most predictive of utilization (Mindel & Wright, 1982).

Another framework for understanding service use is one that examines the factors contributing to a perceived need for help and subsequent service utilization (Yeatts, Crow, & Folts, 1992). In this model the barriers to service are addressed according to three conditions: a) knowledge of services, of procedures, of need; b) access; c) intent as defined by service attractiveness, cultural differences, and attitudes toward service use. Using this framework, service providers can locate where barriers to utilization occur and develop strategies to overcome them.

Wallace (1990) presents a model of service utilization that focuses on service availability, accessibility, and acceptability. Obstacles in any of the three areas can severely jeopardize a program's effectiveness in reaching intended clients. Availability pertains to the presence of programs, and accessibility is the ease with which services can be utilized. Acceptability is the degree to which services and staff are perceived by clients as compatible with their needs and values.

In examining the use services, it is important to also examine persons' patterns of self-care in managing their disabilities and coping with their environments. In one study of older persons in the community, 10% were found to have made some household adjustments that facilitated their ability to live independently, including installation of extra handrails, specially equipped telephones, and modification of bathrooms. The greater the number and severity of the disabilities, the more modifications were made (Struyk & Katsura, 1988).

Other research (Norburn et al., 1995) suggests that the extent of disability is the best predictor of the use of mobility-enhancing strategies and/or equipment. The most common strategy used by impaired older adults is changing behavior, such as doing things less often and more slowly, avoiding lifting heavy objects, and stocking up on items when shopping. Moreover, these self-care strategies are most likely to be found among older persons living alone.

Although having the greatest needs for assistance, the functionally impaired elderly may be among the most difficult to reach. These persons are often isolated in the community and lack appropriate links to services. Without adequate information and knowledge of services and without others to act as liaisons for them, they are at risk of remaining outside of the service system. Moreover, for some persons, the use of any services may be perceived as a first step toward dependency and the loss of autonomy. Rather than seek assistance, which would reflect their incapacity, they prefer to cope on their own.

Understanding the utilization process is basic to meeting the needs of functionally impaired older adults in the community. Effective planning requires comprehensive and inclusive data. Prerequisite to such planning is understanding the specific services that persons want, the factors that contribute to their use of services, and their utilization patterns. In order to further facilitate the attractiveness of services, persons must be assured that actual use is not an indicator of fragility or perceived as the precursor of further dependency.

Community services will be examined according to the general schema of access, home-based, community-based, supportive, and protective. As discussed earlier, the boundaries between these categories are not definitive since one program can encompass more than one role. Neither does the classification provide a continuum of frailty since home-based and community programs may each serve varying levels of impairment.

ACCESS SERVICES

Access services are vital to the care of older persons, as they link them and the services they need. They are the entry points into the service system and are therefore critical to subsequent utilization. Although generally considered part of the service network, access is also obtained through various information channels including the media. Newspapers, television, and the radio can be particularly important sources of access for the more isolated impaired older person who lacks immediate informal supports.

The internet can also be significant in facilitating access to services, as a multitude of websites have been developed that describe programs at both local and national levels. As increasing numbers of older persons are skilled in the use of computers, they may play an even more pivotal role in providing persons with information and even referrals to services. The federal government provides information about community services throughout the country. Programs have also been developed that assess a person's eligibility for services and provide information about available programs within their community. As computers become more available in public libraries and senior centers they can play a major role in linking persons with agencies.

Information and Referral

Information and referral services offer direct links between those requesting services and programs that can address their needs. Information and referral programs are offered by telephone or in person at senior centers, nutrition sites, social service agencies, hospitals, and many private agencies. Providing accurate information is essential, as it can be central in determining whether a person is able to remain in the community. In fact, discerning the array of possible services may be easier for those with lower incomes who are part of the Medicaid program and for whom information and referral services may be most readily available. Those without any public support are often without any accessible entry point into the service system.

Most states have developed their own long-term care information and assistance systems, available to persons of all incomes. However, these programs vary in their effectiveness (Reinhard & Scala, 2001). The most effective statewide programs are those that have strong leadership, a clear plan, adequate funding, and continual promotion.

Some state programs offer services such as case management or planning for older adults. This is often free for those on Medicaid, while those with higher incomes may be required to pay on a sliding fee scale. The effectiveness of this model is debatable, because although the use of Medicaid can help states to meets program costs, it may also deter persons from using the service.

Another concern with these programs is the quality of the staff. Generally there are no credentials for staff and training requirements are not standardized. Consequently, effectiveness can be compromised if persons providing information are not sufficiently knowledgeable, or lack the sensitivity and empathy necessary to work with an impaired older adult. Moreover, few programs follow through on referrals as the primary focus is providing information.

Transportation

Accessing services is difficult if not impossible without adequate transportation. However, the nature of the impairments often precludes older persons' use of either public or private transportation without supports and assistance. At the same time, without appropriate transportation, many are at risk of losing their independence. The ability to use programs and services as well as to engage in preventive care is dependent on transportation.

Efforts to meet the transportation needs of those with impairments can be traced to the amendments made in 1970 to the Urban Mass Transit Act of 1964. These assured that funds would be allocated for the purpose of modifying transportation for the frail and disabled, and ensuring that new transportation be accessible. Subsequent legislation, the National Mass Transportation Assistance Act of 1974 and the 1978 Surface Transportation Assistance Act, provided reduced fares to the elderly and handicapped as well as federal support to programs in nonurban areas.

More recent legislation, the Transportation for Elderly and Handicapped Persons Act of 2001, provides grants to states to further increase accessibility through the purchasing of vehicles and the installation of assistive devices and wheelchair lifts. In addition, grants are given for contracts with private non-profit organizations to enable further development of special services for the elderly and disabled through the Department of Transportation's Elderly Persons with Disabilities Program. Consequently, there exists a vast array of transportation programs at local, state, and federal levels. One of the key issues associated with these programs is their coordination. In 1986 the Department of Health and Human Services and the Department of Transportation, in an attempt to rectify some of the problems besieging the transportation system, formed a Coordinating Council to oversee transportation programs, support local specialized human services coordination, and develop demonstration programs.

The Federal Transit Administration (FTA) within the Department of Transportation is responsible for most funding of programs for older persons and the disabled. In conjunction with the Administration on Aging, the two organizations have begun developing a plan to increase coordination and thus facilitate access to transportation for the elderly and disabled. Their plan involves collecting data regarding all transportation services, developing a joint plan to provide technical assistance to local agencies, working with local agencies to identify barriers and solutions to accessing transportation services, and coordinating the funding among services.

As the number of persons requiring transportation assistance can be expected to increase, adequate funding to meet the needs of this population remains a primary concern. Assuring that programs are given flexibility to design transportation according to the specific needs of their area, and that effective innovative programs are supported and shared can further contribute to the development of services that foster the ability to remain in the community.

Case Management

Case management, which links persons with services and coordinates their care, plays a major role in facilitating service access. The key services provided through case management are assessment, care planning, service arrangement, and monitoring. In addition, the case manager, usually a social worker or a nurse, also acts as the client's advocate in the community.

Case management is offered by a variety of agencies including home nursing programs, social service agencies, and private agencies. The common uniforming goal of the programs is to prevent unnecessary institutionalization of the impaired older person through the provision of services and assistance in the community. The process begins with a comprehensive assessment that usually evaluates the physical, mental, social, and financial status of the applicant. In addition, it reviews the support network of available informal care.

Critical to effective case management is the individualized care plan that should be made in conjunction with the older person and the family, if possible. The plan should serve to supplement existing skills and levels of assistance rather than supplant them. A sensitive care plan provides a basis for enhancing independence and the functioning of the older adult.

Coordinating and monitoring services are the next phases of case management. Coordination can be a sensitive task, in that the manager may assume responsibilities that either the client or the family should be performing. By doing too much, the manager may undermine the capability of the client, while doing too little may mean that needs are not met. Monitoring activities should be associated with the impairment level of the client and the involvement of informal caregivers. In order to assure that changing needs are accommodated, monitoring should be done on a regular basis.

Advocating for clients is a further function of case managers (Rothman & Sager, 1998). In this role, managers can help to assure that individual clients obtain specific services or benefits. Advocating takes on a larger role as managers focus on changes in the community to foster the development of resources, or to assure the further coordination of programs.

Under the Medicaid waiver programs, many states have initiated care management programs for frail older adults and the disabled. In some states the managers are employed by public services; in others they are contract employees from other agencies. With variations among programs, eligibility criteria, services offered, and resources, it is difficult to establish the overall effectiveness in case management in enabling older impaired persons to maintain their independence. Some studies have found no effect on the quality of life of recipients (Gagnon, Schein, & McVey, 1999), while others have found that programs prevent disability and institutionalization (Stuck et al., 1995; Shapiro & Taylor, 2002).

One of the major criticisms of case management is that it lays another layer of service on an already fragmented long-term care system, rather than focusing attention on altering the system (Callahan, 1989). Case management acts as a response to the needs of the system rather than to the needs of the elderly. Other concerns revolve around a lack of guidelines, training requirements, or standards for case management.

The services may or may not be offered by licensed professionals, and even the professionals may not have any specific background in case management Without certification requirements for case management, any person can define himself or herself as a geriatric case manager and provide services. A further issue is the conflict of interests that can arise if agencies providing direct services, such as home care, also offer case management.

The role of case management in the delivery of community care continues to expand. Given this growth, it becomes imperative to assure that the providers themselves are qualified and that there are sufficient services and resources to coordinate. The role of case managers as advocates is often overlooked, and yet it may be in this role that they can have the greatest impact on the community. Given their direct contact with older adults, they are often in the position of recognizing gaps in services and linkages, as well as those programs most often denying benefits. Using this knowledge, case managers can work to address system problems that further impede the well-being of older adults in the community.

HOME-BASED SERVICES

Home-based services assist functionally impaired older persons with their activities of daily living and household management. Such services include home health care that provides assistance with medications, wounds, specific therapies, and activities of daily living; and homemaker services that focus on household tasks, help with grooming, and physical care. Whereas home health care is provided by nurses, other services are offered by home attendants or home health aides under the supervision of a home health or social service agency. Services for older adults are funded under a variety of public programs including Medicare, Medicaid, Veterans Administration, Title XX programs, and the Older Americans Act.

Home Care

Following a rapid growth in home health care services in the 1990s, the Balanced Budget Act of 1997 restrained services by initiating a prospective payment system to agencies, and a system of diagnostic related groupings for patient care with payments based on 60-day periods. Subsequently, many agencies closed or did not accept Medicare beneficiaries.

Under Medicare, home care services for impaired older adults are restricted to those who are homebound and require skilled services; that is, physical therapy, speech therapy, occupational therapy, and skilled nursing. There are no limitations on the length of care, but care plans must be authorized by a physician and reviewed every 60 days. However, the role that the benefit plays in meeting the chronic needs of many functionally impaired elderly who do not require skilled care but who do require ongoing assistance to remain at home remains debatable. Moreover, the closure of many agencies means that services are not necessarily available, and that existing agencies may be reluctant to accept patients with greater care needs whose reimbursement may be more doubtful.

Medicaid home care is offered under the traditional state Medicaid programs to low-income elderly, as well as through waiver programs to persons who would qualify for nursing home placement. Comparable to Medicare, care plans must be directed by a physician and reviewed every 60 days. However, there are no requirements regarding skilled care or whether the person is homebound. States may also offer personal care services to beneficiaries that include all services that help with activities of daily living but are not dependent on skilled care. Within federal guidelines, states decide on the amount and extent of services to be offered on deductibles and copayments.

Many Medicaid programs have been innovative in their design of home care services for impaired older adults since they are perceived as primary mechanisms for reducing the nursing home population, and thus reducing costs associated with long-term care. However, as states wrestle with increasing expenditures and decreasing budgets, programs—which are not often seen as a priority—remain very vulnerable.

Home-Delivered Meals

Home-delivered meals, provided through private non-profit organizations or nutrition programs under the Older Americans Act, can be a critical resource in helping older persons stay in the community. As well as providing meals, the staff and volunteers of the programs can offer emotional support to the homebound, and serve as links to other services.

Most of the 15,000 nutrition sites provide home-delivered meals to the elderly. Moreover, these sites have seen a gradual shift from congregate meals to more home-delivered meals. A national survey of nutrition programs funded through the Older Americans Act reports a continued transfer from congregate meal programs to home-delivered meals (Administration on Aging, 2003), with almost all providers expecting the increase to continue. Underscoring the need for the programs is the fact that nearly 40% of home delivery programs have waiting lists. State agencies speculate that this is due to participants aging and becoming frailer, unmet transportation needs, and a growing number of persons living alone.

Studies are also being made to help improve the targeting of home-delivered meals to those most at risk in the community for functional decline. Factors such as weight change and medication use as well as disability have been used as indicators of need (Sharkey, Haines, & Zohoori, 2000; Sharkey, 2002). The use of medications, difficulties in shopping for food, inadequate income, and difficulty preparing food place older persons at risk of poor nutrition and increased severity of disability.

COMMUNITY-BASED PROGRAMS

Community-based programs serve older adults in congregate settings and provide care for those who are unimpaired to those who are extremely impaired. A major advantage to congregate programs is the opportunity for socialization and interaction with peers that is usually lacking in home-based settings. Such activities can be particularly important to the older person whose needs for mental and social stimulation can be overlooked in efforts to meet demands associated with physical function.

Nutrition Programs

Nutrition programs were formally authorized under the Older Americans Act of 1973 to provide at least one hot meal a day in a congregate setting to all persons over the age of 60 years. The original goals of the program were to improve the health of seniors and to increase social interaction. At the same time, the programs were intended to foster independence by offering counseling and referrals to other social services, and to offer screening, assessment, and nutrition counseling. From their beginning, the programs sought to serve the more frail and vulnerable in the community, and continue to target those at risk of losing their independence. Nutrition sites include schools, churches, and senior centers. Funding for the programs comes from Title III of the Older Americans Act, participant contributions, and local donations.

An evaluation of the program in 1996 (Administration on Aging, 1996) found that 80%–90% of the participants had incomes 200% below the poverty level, with twice as many as the overall elderly population living alone and having weight problems that placed them at risk for further chronic illness. The meals were found to increase the dietary intakes of the participants and helped to meet their nutritional needs, while decreasing their social isolation. Providing program transportation, having longer hours, and offering meals 7 days a week can further strengthen the role of nutrition programs in meeting the needs of older persons.

Senior Centers

Senior centers have continued to play a major role in the network of community-based services since their beginnings in the 1940s. The first centers focused on socialization activities for seniors who were well functioning but who might be experiencing the loneliness and isolation that frequently accompanies the aging process. Centers continue to be one of the most utilized of all programs for the elderly, with approximately 10 million older adults participating at 12,000 senior centers across the country (Beisgen & Kraitchman, 2003).

Early descriptions of senior center participants describe them as being older, active, and relatively healthy. Centers in general have been viewed as maintaining their original focus on the well elderly and therefore have failed to target the minority, low-income, and frail population (Krout, Cutler, & Coward, 1990). Moreover, to focus on these groups may affect the ability of centers to attract and retain their current well participants (Ralston, 1991). At the same time, as participants have begun to age, centers may be required to change focus.

The capacity of centers to provide services for functionally impaired older adults remains in question. A study of senior centers in New York State found that directors felt it would be difficult to effectively integrate a high proportion of frail persons into their programs (Cox & Monk, 1989). It was easier to integrate those with physical impairments than those with behavioral or emotional ones. Center directors saw their participants as more accepting of established members who became frail than of those who were frail when they joined. Data from the centers also revealed that the proportion of well participants significantly decreased as the proportion of frail participants increased.

Overall, findings indicated that both staff and the well participants were reluctant to integrate. Thus, although the majority of center directors stated that they had formal guidelines for serving impaired older persons, few had actually developed programs specific to their needs. Few centers made their own assessments of the impairment levels, most being based on referrals from other agencies, and very few based on medical screenings. Consequently, the extent to which a supposedly frail individual could actually participate was not evaluated on-site.

The centers with the highest proportions of frail participants were those with specially trained staff and those with programs coordinated with other agencies. The expertise of these staff and the links with other services promoted integration, though it was not clear whether the training and coordination preceded or followed the increase in frail participants.

Subsequent reviews of centers (Krout, 1995, 1996) find that 5%–10% of persons attending centers are vision- or hearing-impaired, frail, or cognitively impaired and that centers are providing some programming for them. However, most of this programming is related to health maintenance, assessments, and referrals rather than actual programs. A further indicator of the difficulties associated with integration is that the frail were brought to these centers in a slow, deliberate manner, so that they were not placed "abruptly" into contact with the well users.

These findings continue to suggest that the ability of centers to serve impaired older adults remains in question. Indeed, without transportation, skilled staff, and special efforts, the complete integration of these older adults into centers remains doubtful. Moreover, as centers begin to focus on programs such as computer skills development, and activities for the functionally well older adults, their abilities to serve those with greater needs remains in question.

Adult Day Care

Adult day care concentrates on serving the functionally impaired by offering a program of health, social, and special support services in a protective setting. Day care can therefore play a significant role in the lives of the frail elderly as it offers support and social interaction, while providing caregivers with respite assistance. Programs usually provide transportation, medical care, health monitoring, and socialization activities. Although programs can serve both physically and cognitively impaired persons, centers are also developing that care for only persons with Alzheimer's disease or other dementias.

Findings from a national survey of adult day care centers reveal that there are 3,407 licensed adult day care centers operating in the United States. The majority of these are non-profit operations (Cox, 2003). The average cost of care is $56 per day, but the average charge is $46 a day, indicating that programs are not meeting their costs. Medicaid and other public programs, including Title XX Social Services Block Grants and funds under Title IIIB of the Older Americans Act, pay for 51% of all costs. Families pay for approximately 47% and long-term care insurance pays for less than 1%. The survey also found that many centers were not fully utilized. This shows a continuing need for more public education and information.

A survey of day care programs identified three models of programs: One stresses rehabilitation, is associated with a nursing home or rehabilitation hospital, and serves the most dependent elderly; a second model is affiliated with a general hospital and serves a less physically frail but often more mentally impaired population; a third model is the special purpose center that serves only one population such as Alzheimer's patients or the mentally ill (Weissert et al., 1989).

Data from Weissert et al.'s survey found that although participants were functionally dependent, they were at low risk of nursing home placement. They were younger than most nursing home patients, less dependent, more likely to be married, and less frequently mentally impaired. Impairment was highest in bathing, grooming, and dressing skills. A review of IADL impairments showed participants required assistance in handling money and shopping. According to program administrators, more than half of participants would require nursing home placement if day care were not available.

In an extensive review of the role of day care, Gaugler and Zarit (2001) found that day care programs did not significantly impact on families delaying institutionalization, but that such reductions can occur if programs target those most at risk of placement. In addition, participants do show some improvements in functioning and families are generally satisfied with the programs. The main benefits of programs seem to be with their immediate psychosocial outcomes for participants and their caregivers—rather than their potential as substitutes for institutional care. At the same time, it is important to consider that these outcomes may be sufficient in themselves.

Day care is apparently serving a different population of frail elderly from those at risk of institutionalization. Critics of the programs may perceive them as additional services that require resources and funds, rather than reducing overall costs. However, using a broader perspective on impairment and its impact on individuals, day care has the potential to play a stabilizing and even preventive role in future expenditures. It affects both participant and caregiver well-being and expands the community options available to impaired older adults.

SUPPORTIVE SERVICES

Supportive services entail a very broad category of programs that assist persons of different impairment levels. Services are often categorized as home- or community-based. Home care, telephone reassurance, and respite care are examples of home-based services. Financial assistance, information, counseling, support groups, and legal services are examples of supportive programs that are offered in a variety of community-based settings. This section discusses examples of home- and community-based supportive services that can be critical in fostering the independence of older adults.

Telephone Reassurance and Friendly Visiting

Both of these home-based support programs provide emotional and practical support to frail elderly in the community. Volunteers, under the supervision of a professional, usually staff the services. Social service agencies, senior centers, and churches are the primary providers of these services.

In telephone reassurance, the elderly participant is telephoned at least once daily. If there is no answer, the volunteer contacts the police or another specified individual who will then visit the home. Additionally, the volunteer can provide both advice and counseling while acting as an important link to other services. However, the ability of the volunteer to do so is closely dependent upon his or her training.

One of the major barriers to program utilization is the attitudes of older adults. Suspiciousness regarding the nature of the service and unfamiliarity with a particular volunteer can deter its use. In addition, research has also indicated that many are not familiar with the program. In one study, it was found that only 31% were informed about telephone reassurance programs, in comparison with 78% who knew about senior centers (Calsyn & Winter, 1999).

Volunteers are also the primary source of staff of friendly visiting programs to the homebound elderly. Again, these individuals can be links to other services while also providing emotional support to those at risk of becoming isolated. These visitors are usually not trained in counseling and are thus expected to limit their services to conversation and leisure activities. In many instances, however, they may be the only ones available to detect marked changes in an older person's condition, changes that could signify a need for more intense assistance.

Respite Care

Respite care provides relief to caregivers and is a key supportive service generally offered in the home. Public funding is available through many state Medicaid programs, for family caregivers of persons with Alzheimer's disease through Title III of the Older Americans Act, and for other caregivers through the Family Caregiver Support Amendment. In addition, many states use general revenue funds to provide respite care.

Respite care can be short-term, provided a few hours a day for a limited period of time, or it can be all day, with the service either provided at home or in a day care program. Some respite programs offer 24-hour care, usually in a hospital or nursing home. In-home respite is the format most desired by caregivers since it causes the least disruption to the older person. It is similar to home care in that the respite worker often assists the individual with functioning or performs household tasks.

Respite care out of the home can permit caregivers to have a longer period of relief. Placement in an institution such as a hospital or nursing home may also be more appropriate for the very impaired frail who require more intensive supervision. However, such services may also be a link to eventual institutional placement of the older patient. In one study of nursing home respite, many of the caregivers used the service as a trial program for institutionalization. Following the temporary placement, they felt less stress and guilt about permanently placing the relative in the nursing home (Miller & Goldman, 1989).

With the focus of respite being on support and relief for the caregiver, studies on the outcomes of respite show varying results. Most studies were conducted on caregivers of relatives with dementia. One review of the literature on respite services found that benefits are actually modest, but that these findings could be due to varying methodological problems in the evaluations and to limited service provision (Zarit, Gaugler, & Jarrott, 1999). A further review of 29 respite studies also found little evidence that respite had any consistent or enduring beneficial effect on caregivers, although 10 of the studies did report improvements in caregiver well-being (McNally, Ben-Shlomo, & Newman, 1999). Conversely, other research (Burns & Rabins, 2000) find relatives reporting that respite is the most important intervention in relieving their stress.

Although it would be logical that respite would be a much sought-after service, like day care, it remains underutilized. In a study of respite services offered in homes, nursing homes, and day care facilities, Montgomery (1988) found that caregivers were difficult to reach and resistant to using the service, even after agreeing to do so and with the service offered free of charge. Of those using the respite, the majority preferred short in-home respite to nursing home or day care. All users were highly satisfied with the programs and interested in using other services such as seminars and support groups.

Another study (Cox, 1997) found that even after going through the application process and being accepted into a program, caregivers may be reluctant to utilize the service. Among those who did use the service, it was relatively late in the caregiving career when the program itself is insufficient to meet the needs of the caregiver or those of the relative. Reaching caregivers at an earlier stage of their caregiving, offering sufficient amounts of respite, and providing them with other interventions that can further strengthen their abilities are potential ways of increasing both utilization and its impact. People will use respite if they understand it, if it is provided in sufficient amounts, and if the aide is reliable and trained (Blume et al., 1990).

To address many of the gaps occurring with respite services, the Life Span Respite Care Act of 2003 has been introduced into Congress for consideration as part of the Public Health Service Act. The act seeks to assure the development of a coordinated community-based system of respite care. The act entails the expansion of respite services to family caregivers, statewide dissemination and coordination of respite services, and improving access to and the quality of the care. The bill requires that service providers monitor and screen respite workers and assure that they have the necessary skills to meet the needs of the care receiver.

Mental Health Counseling

As older adults encounter the challenges of aging, particularly those accompanying physical impairments and limitations, they are vulnerable to experiencing feelings of loss and depression. Often persons adapt to the negative effects of aging by narrowing the focus of their lives to those domains in which they are still successful, and using those domains to compensate for other losses, a process called "selective optimizing" (Baltes & Baltes, 1990). Certainly, persons will vary in their ability to make such compensations. To the extent that they are unable to cope, the feelings of loss may further undermine their well-being.

Mental health counseling is a critical community support service that can assist persons in their adaptation to the transitions accompanying aging. Unfortunately, mental health services for older adults remain poorly funded and fragmented (Gatz & Smyer, 2001). The use of services by older persons is dramatically less than that of other population groups, with fewer than 3% of those over 65 receiving outpatient mental health treatment by a specialist (Olfson & Pincus, 1996). Concurrently, about 15% of persons over age 65 report having severe depressive symptoms, with this proportion increasing to over 20% of those 80 and older (Health and Retirement Study, 1998).

There are potential barriers to the use of mental health counseling by older adults. These include feelings of stigma associated with mental health problems, attitudes of providers that little can be done, a lack of access to qualified providers, and financing issues. Medicare does not give parity in its payments to mental health providers, meaning that older adults must pay for a larger portion of the care themselves. In addition, private health insurance policies offer only limited coverage. Under Medicaid, states have the option of what types of mental health services to provide, while reimbursement rates to providers are usually less than those of other insurers (Administration on Aging, 2001).

Consequently, when persons do seek mental health care, it is usually from their primary care physician. The ability of these professionals to accurately diagnose and treat the problems of these patients is dependent upon their interest and skill. However, it is important to note that less than 3% of all medical students take one course in geriatrics and only three medical schools in the country require a geriatric rotation for medical students (O'Neill & Barry, 2003). Thus, physicians are not trained to recognize or understand the complex issues confronting older patients or their underlying psychological needs.

Another barrier to mental health care is the lack of trained geriatric mental health professionals such as geropsychiatrists, geropsychologists, and geriatric social workers. These shortages are expected to become most noticeable as the size of the older population and their need for mental health services continue to grow, resulting in a major public health problem (Bartels & Smyer, 2002). Without direct interventions that increase the numbers of mental health professionals skilled in the counseling of older adults, many older persons will continue to struggle with feelings of depression and loss.

PROTECTIVE SERVICES

Protective services are designed to assure that the rights and benefits available to older adults are protected. Given the maze of programs designed to address their needs, these services serve as advocates on elders' behalf, to ensure protection of their interests.

Providing legal assistance to the elderly was made a priority service under the 1975 amendments to the Older Americans Act. Since 1981, local Area Agencies on Aging have been required to spend a percentage of their funding on legal assistance for the vulnerable elderly. Further emphasis on the need for protection of elder rights was made in 1992 with the establishment of Title VII of the act, Allotments for Vulnerable Elder Rights Activities.

The 1992 amendment combined the ombudsman program, elder abuse and exploitations programs, and legal assistance programs into one, in an effort to increase coordination in each state. Every state now has a legal assistance developer whose role is to develop legal and advocacy assistance for the most vulnerable elderly. The Administration on Aging has also developed legal hotlines staffed by trained volunteers who can answer many legal questions and refer persons to local attorneys who provide pro bono or reduced-fee consultation.

The Commission on Legal Problems of the Elderly of the American Bar Association focuses on the rights of older persons and conducts research into a range of topics that affect the lives of these persons. Reflective of the many dimensions of the problems affecting the interests of the older population, the commission is composed of professionals from the fields of law, health, and social services. Policy papers on topics such as elder abuse, guardianship, home care, Social Security, legal rights, and housing have been issued.

The National Senior Citizens Law Center was established in 1972 and acts as an advocacy organization for the rights of older low-income persons and those with disabilities. Among the issues it is involved in are the protection of state Medicaid programs and long-term care services and their development, and standards for assisted living programs. The Center also provides training to local advocates to assure optimal representation of elderly clients.

Elder Abuse

Elder abuse is the most extreme infraction of the rights of older persons. Those dependent on others to meet their needs (the frail) are clearly the most vulnerable. Included in the definitions of abuse are financial exploitation, sexual abuse, physical abuse, psychological abuse, and neglect. Neglect can be by the caregiver, but also includes self-neglect when the older person is not sufficiently caring for his or her own needs. The National Center for Elder Abuse, a program funded through the Administration on Aging, acts as a resource for public and private agencies and individuals regarding training and assistance in elder abuse.

Every state has elder abuse reporting laws and systems although there are variations among them. In most states, adult protective services are responsible for investigating suspected cases of abuse or neglect. However, concerns continue regarding the effectiveness of these programs in addressing the problem. A 1996 national study of abuse found that cases are still seriously underreported; for every one case reported to adult protective services, five were unreported (National Center on Elder Abuse, 1998). Rates of abuse and neglect were highest for older women with the majority of perpetrators being relatives or spouses.

Given the extent of the problem, it is troubling that funding for elder abuse prevention programs has remained constant, slightly over $5 million a year, since the early 1990s. At the state levels, adult protective services receive much less funding than those for child protection. Consequently, the ability of these services to develop effective interventions that reduce elders' risks for abuse and neglect are seriously compromised.

SUMMARY

A wide array of services are in place that can have a significant impact in addressing the care of older persons in the community. These services offer a continuum of assistance, depending on the needs of the person, and may be offered in either the home or the community. However, gaps between services continue and limited resources preclude equal access. In addition, many individual and structural barriers can affect a person's use of services. Understanding these barriers and the way they can impact utilization is a prerequisite for effectiveness in serving older persons.

Limited resources are a problem for most community programs, with the demand for services often exceeding the supply. At the same time, having limited resources means that many programs must depend on volunteers or on staff who are not necessarily trained in gerontology. This reality is in itself a major concern.

Responsive systems of community care must be both comprehensive and coordinated in order to best meet the needs of the population. In addition, services must be attractive to the older population that they seek to serve. To the extent that they are associated with stigma or dependency, they are vulnerable to being underutilized. To be most effective, services must offer options and assistance tailored to individual needs. Such a process necessitates knowledge and understanding of the ways that persons perceive their own limitations, problems, and the services intended to assist them. Most importantly, community care demands a commitment by policymakers and providers if it is to assume the weighty role of service provider.

REFERENCES

Administration on Aging. (1996). *Nutrition evaluation report: Program funding, costs, and efficiency.* Rockville, MD: Department of Health and Human Services.
Administration on Aging. (2001). *Older adults and mental health: Issues and opportunities.* Rockville, MD: Department of Health and Human Services.

Administration on Aging. (2003). *The elderly nutrition program.* Rockville, MD: Department of Health and Human Services.

Anderson, R., & Newman, J. (1973). Societal and individual determinants of medical care utilization in the United States. *Milbank Memorial Fund Quarterly, 51,* 95–124.

Baltes, P., & Baltes, M. (1990). Psychological perspectives on successful aging: The model of selective optimization with compensation. In P. B. Baltes & M. M. Baltes (Eds.), *Successful aging* (pp. 1–36). Cambridge, UK: University of Cambridge Press.

Bartels, S., & Smyer, M. (2002). Mental disorders of aging: An emerging public health crisis? *Generations, 26,* 14–20.

Beisgen, B., & Kraitchman, M. (2003). *Senior centers: Opportunities for successful aging.* New York: Springer Publishing.

Blume, L., Persily, N., Mirones, M., Swaby-Thorne, A., & Albury, S. (1990). Anatomy of the Alzheimer's respite care program (ARCP). *Home Health Care Services Quarterly, 11,* 75–90.

Burns, A., & Rabins, P. (2000). Carer burden in dementia. *International Journal of Geriatric Psychiatry, 15,* S9–S13.

Callahan, J. J. (1989). Case management for the elderly: A panacea? *Journal of Aging and Social Policy, 1*(1/2), 181–195.

Calsyn, R., & Winter, J. (1999). Predicting specific service awareness dimensions. *Research on Aging, 21,* 761–780.

Cox, C. (1997). Findings from a statewide program of respite use: A comparison of program users, stoppers, and non-users. *Gerontologist, 37,* 511–517.

Cox, C., & Monk, A. (1989). Integrating the frail and well elderly: The experience of senior centers. *Journal of Gerontological Social Work, 15,* 131–144.

Cox, N. (2003, March). *A national study of adult day care services.* Paper presented at the Joint Conferences of the American Society on Aging and National Council on the Aging, Chicago.

Gagnon, A., Schein, C., & McVey, L. (1999). Randomized controlled trial of nurse case management of frail older people. *Journal of the American Geriatrics Society, 47,* 1118–1124.

Gatz, M., & Smyer, M. (2001). Mental health and aging at the onset of the twenty-first century. In J. Birren & K. Schaie (Eds.), *Handbook of the psychology of aging* (5th ed.). San Diego: Academic Press.

Gerontological Society of America. (1978). *Working with older people: A guide to practice.* Rockville, MD: U.S. Department of Health, Education, and Welfare.

Googler, J., & Zarit, S. (2001). The effectiveness of adult day services for disabled older people. *Journal of Aging and Social Policy, 12*(2), 23–47.

Health and Retirement Study (HRS). (1998). Ann Arbor: University of Michigan, Michigan Institute for Social Research.

Krout, J. (1995). Senior centers and services for the frail elderly. *Journal of Aging and Social Policy, 7,* 59–76.

Krout, J. (1996). Senior center programming and frailty among older persons. *Journal of Gerontological Social Work, 26,* 19–34.

Krout, J., Cutler, S., & Coward, R. (1990). Correlates of senior center participation: A national analysis. *Gerontologist, 30*(1), 172–179.

McNally, S., Ben-Shlomo, Y., & Newman, S. (1999). Effects of respite care on informal carers' well-being: A systematic review. *Disability and Rehabilitation, 21,* 1–14.

Miller, D., & Goldman, L. (1989). Perceptions of caregivers about special respite services for the elderly. *Gerontologist, 29,* 408–410.

Mindel, C., & Wright, R. (1982). The use of social services by black and white elderly: The role of social support systems. *Journal of Gerontological Social Work, 4,* 106–125.

Monk, A. (1990). Gerontological social services. In A. Monk (Ed.), *Handbook of gerontological social services* (2nd ed.). New York: Columbia University Press.

Montgomery, R. (1988). Respite care: Lessons from a controlled design study. *Health Care Financing Review,* Supplement, 133–138.

National Center for Elder Abuse. (1998). *The 1998 national elder abuse incidence study.* Washington, DC: Author.

Norburn, J., Bernard, S., Konrad, T., Woomert, A., DeFriese, G., Kalsbeek, W., Koch, G., & Ory, M. (1995). Self-care and assistance from others in coping with functional status limitations among a national sample of older adults. *Journal of Gerontology, Social Sciences, 50B,* S101–S109.

Olfson, M., & Pincus, H. (1996). Outpatient mental health care in non-hospital settings: Distribution of patients across provider groups. *American Journal of Psychiatry, 153,* 1353–1356.

O'Neill, G., & Barry, P. (2003). Training physicians in geriatric care: Responding to critical need. *Public Policy and Aging Report, 13*(2), 17–21. Washington, DC: Gerontology Society of America.

Reinhard, S., & Scala, M. (2001). *Navigating the long term care maze: New approaches to information in three states.* Washington, DC: Public Policy Institute, American Association of Retired Persons.

Rothman, J., & Sager, J. (1998). *Case management: Integrating individual and community practice* (2nd ed.). Boston: Allyn & Bacon.

Shapiro, A., & Taylor, M. (2002). Effects of a community-based early intervention program on the subjective well-being, institutionalization, and mortality of low income elders. *Gerontologist, 42,* 334–341.

Sharkey, J. (2002). The interrelationship of nutritional risk factors, indicators of nutritional risk, and severity of disability among home-delivered meal participants. *Gerontologist, 42,* 373–380.

Sharkey, J., Haines, P., & Zohoori, N. (2000). Community-based screening: Association between nutritional risk and severe functional disability among rural home-delivered nutrition participants. *Journal of Nutrition for the Elderly, 20,* 1–15.

Skinner, J. (1990). Federal programs for the vulnerable aged. In Z. Harel, P. l. Ehrlich, & R. Hubbard (Eds.), *The vulnerable aged: People, services and policies.* New York: Springer Publishing.

Struyk, R., & Katsora, H. (1988). *Aging at home: How the elderly adjust their housing without moving.* New York: Haworth Press.

Stuck, A., Aronow, H., Steiner, A., Alessi, C., Bula, C., Gold, M., Yukas, K., Nisenbaum, R., Rubenstein, L., & Beck, J. (1995). A trial of in-home comprehensive geriatric assessments for elderly people living in the community. *New England Journal of Medicine, 333,* 1184–1189.

Tobin, S., & Toseland, R. (1990). Models of services for the elderly. In A. Monk (Ed.), *Handbook of gerontological social services* (pp. 27–51). New York: Columbia University Press.

Wallace, S. (1990). The no-care zone: Availability, accessibility, and acceptability in community based long term care. *Gerontologist, 30,* 254–262.

Weissert, W. G., Elston, J. M., Bolda, E. J., Cready, C. M., Zelma, W. N., Sloane, P. D., Kalsbee, W. D., Mutran, E., Rice, T. H., & Koch, G. G. (1989). Models of adult day care: Findings from a national survey. *Gerontologist, 5,* 640–649.

Yeatts, D., Crow, T., & Folts, E. (1992). Service use among low-income minority elderly: Strategies for overcoming barriers. *Gerontologist, 32,* 24–31.

Zarit, S., Gaugler, J., & Jarrott, S. (1999). Useful services for families: Research findings and directions. *International Journal of Geriatric Psychiatry, 14,* 165–181.

Chapter 5

Housing Needs and Responses

Essential to remaining in the community is housing responsive to the needs of older persons with impairments. Independent living is predicated upon residing in an environment that is compatible with the individual's functional status, that is, compensatory for their limitations and supportive of their abilities. The nature of the physical environment is fundamental in determining whether a person with limitations is able to function in his or her own home. Concomitantly, the level of functioning indicates the types of modifications that may be required to maintain the person's independence and even prevent further deterioration.

Housing can play a significant role in the health outcomes of the disabled elderly (Newman, 2003). As older persons with limitations spend more time in the home, they are particularly sensitive to its physical condition and are at additional risk for accidents if this is inadequate. With services delivered in the home, the setting can affect what is provided and even the feasibility of offering services. In addition, neighborhood safety concerns can affect the ability of the older person to leave the home as well as the inclination of providers to provide care.

Special adaptations and assistive devices, as well as support services, can provide the resources enabling seniors to remain independent. Moreover, targeted services such as information on contractors or knowing exactly what house modifications are needed may be more important than income in determining whether changes are made (Struyk & Katsura, 1988). Other research (Pynoos, 1993) suggests that many persons are unaware of the usefulness of home modifications, and that affordability and inaccessibility due to poor service systems can act as barriers.

When the environment becomes unmanageable to the older person, the only option may be moving. A decision to move may be based on the inaccessibility of resources needed for home adaptations, rather than the level of impairment or functioning. A survey of over 2,000 older persons found that the majority would like to stay in their homes as long as possible, and resist the idea of moving, with over 70% of those able to do so having made some home modification. The most frequent modifications included installing light switches in stairwells and adding grab bars or handrails in bathrooms or stairwells (AARP, 2000).

HOUSING CONDITIONS OF IMPAIRED OLDER PERSONS

Using data from the American Housing Survey (AHS), Newman (2003) found that approximately 14% of older persons in the community have housing-related disabilities, according to their own reports of difficulty in functioning or their need for assistance. Most of these difficulties were due to mobility problems, housework or laundry, bathing, preparing and cooking food, and reaching bathroom facilities.

Approximately half of those surveyed lived in a home that had some assistive modification, while 23% reported unmet needs for such modifications. In comparison to those without such needs, these 23% were more likely to be Black, female, living alone, receiving public assistance, and having very low income. They were also more likely to live in older housing in poorer neighborhoods, to rent, and to pay lower rents than the nondisabled elderly. The data also indicate an increase in home modifications between 1978 and 1995 with a corresponding decrease in unmet needs. The most common modifications were additions of ramps, handrails, grab bars, and accessible bathrooms. Among the reported unmet needs were extra-wide doors or hallways, modified wall sockets, modified faucets or cabinets, and door handles instead of knobs.

Using data from the same American Housing Survey, Louie (1999) found that approximately three out of four older adults with disabilities who reported a need for some modification in their home had at least one modification already. However, only half reported having the specific modification that they needed. Whereas 49% with mobility difficulties affecting their ability to enter the home had some assistive modification, only 15% having difficulties in the kitchen had any type of modification. Consequently, even with adjustments made, many impaired older persons still find their housing not amenable to their function levels.

It is important to note, however, that in some instances adaptations are actually resisted. Many elderly reject devices that would identify them as "disabled" (Christenson, 1990). Research (Mathieson, Kronefeld, & Keith, 2002) has also found that the most impaired elderly are less likely to make modifications in their homes than the less impaired, suggesting that once a certain level of impairment (e.g., becoming bedridden or having severe mobility problems) is reached, the person is less likely to make changes in the home. Having supplemental health insurance was also found to increase the likelihood of making home adaptations enabling persons to remain independent.

PROVISIONS FOR STAYING IN THE HOME

Home Repair and Home Adaptation Programs

Older persons tend to live in homes that need repair. Over 60% live in homes over 20 years old. Making repairs to these houses is often beyond the capacity of the frail householder. In addition, attending to the routine maintenance of a home, repairing a gutter or broken windows, mowing the lawn, and unclogging a toilet are chores that can be impossible for the frail to complete. Elders' inability to complete or obtain assistance for these tasks, although generally inexpensive and requiring little expertise, gives many older persons no choice but to move.

Funds for home repairs are available from various federal, state, and local sources. In addition, many communities have developed cadres of volunteers who routinely assist the elderly with these tasks. However, as noted by Pynoos (1992), the absence of any national program, along with the gaps in the current system, leave many elderly unable to obtain assistance.

The Farmer's Home Administration provides loans to low-income elderly in rural areas for assistance in removing health or safety hazards, or bringing a home up to established standards. Loans for home repairs are also available to low-income elderly through the Department of Housing and Urban Development. As with all government programs, though, the availability of such funds fluctuates, compromising the real impact they might have on the elderlys' housing needs.

Assistance with minor repairs and routine maintenance is also offered through many local Area Agencies on Aging with funding from the Older Americans Act (OAA) and block grants. The services under OAA, however, are not mandated and are therefore not uniformly available throughout the country. Block grant funding is likely to go to specific neighborhoods and is not necessarily allocated to the elderly.

Since the preference of most elderly people is to remain in their own homes, it is important to examine what accommodations may be necessary in order to make homes adaptable to their needs. Assistance with household and personal care is only one type of intervention that may be required. In addition, changes may be necessary in the actual structure of the house. Lowering sinks, widening hallways for wheelchair accessibility, having bathrooms on the first floor, and installing ramps are some of these kinds of adaptations.

Programs and services to adapt homes to the needs of the frail are very limited. In most instances, elderly homeowners must pay privately for modifications, though some loans are offered through government programs. The scarcity of these funds, however, means that adaptations are not routinely made. Some communities enlist volunteers (e.g., students or other community groups) to perform repairs or modifications. However, maintaining a core group of skilled volunteers that can adequately meet the needs of a community's aging population is difficult.

A survey of home repair and modification programs in 23 cities in the United States found that all the cities had programs to assist older people, with most not requiring any contributions for their services. However, most programs did not target older persons or focus on meeting their needs. The most common repairs of those that did target the elderly were for electrical, plumbing, and heating and cooling systems, with roof repair and replacement the next most frequently performed repair (Gaberlavage & Forsythe, 1995). The findings from the study suggest that the focus was on maintaining property rather than making specific modifications that addressed the needs of disabled elders.

Assistive Technology

Home adaptations are not limited to structural or assistive devices. The application of technological advances has made the home more accommodating to the frail individual. Telephones, one of the most common technological devices found in the home, can be particularly vital to older impaired persons. Telephones link them with services as well as social contacts. For many, however, using a telephone can be challenging. Vision impairment may make it difficult to read numbers, mobility problems may make answering the phone challenging, arthritis can inhibit a person's ability to dial and hold the receiver, and hearing impairments can act as barriers to hearing the ring or the caller's voice.

Advances in telecommunications have addressed many of these problems. Telephones can be equipped with amplifiers and speakers to increase the volume of the ring and the voice, large numbers and letters are available to assist with dialing, and cordless phones can be important for those with mobility limitations. Telephones with memories that allow numbers to be dialed by pushing only one button, and may even include pictures of the person to be called, can facilitate use by those with physical and even cognitive impairments.

Personal Emergency Response Systems (PERS) are devices that can attend to emergencies, such as falls, that might occur in the home. They can provide a sense of security to persons living alone and their caregivers. The system includes a small radio transmitter, worn as a bracelet or around the neck, that transmits a telephone signal to a 24-hour emergency center when help is needed. The person does not need to be at home to make the transmission. Systems are also available that automatically call the center if no activity has been noted in a particular period of time. The response centers may be in hospitals or run by private companies. Friends, relatives, or a formal agency, identified by the user, are contacted by the response center as soon as an emergency signal is received.

There is some evidence that users of the system appear to be able to use it as a substitute for home care. As such, it can significantly reduce costs for the frail elderly. An evaluation of PERS's ability to replace home attendants was made by giving the device to 54 clients in a Medicaid-funded home health care program matched with a control group who did not receive the device (Coordinated Care Management Corporation, 1989). Both groups had impaired functioning with the majority of each eligible for residence in a health-related facility. The results of the 25-month study found no differences in functioning between the groups, but the PERS users used fewer hours of home care, resulting in a large cost savings to the program. The majority of clients felt secure with the system and reported that it increased their independence.

The services can foster the independence of older impaired persons, but only a small percentage of those who could benefit from the service actually have it. Factors affecting its use are cost and the individual's denial of need (Mann, 1997). Although the service is available in some states under the Medicaid waiver programs, others must pay for it privately, and for those on limited incomes the monthly cost can be prohibitive. Psychological factors may also inhibit use of the system, as they may be perceived as symbols of limitations and dependency or as impinging on privacy.

As the century begins and innovations continue to develop, the scope of devices that can assist the impaired elderly continues to expand. As well as offering relief, assistive technology is important in that it can also foster a personal sense of control and self-confidence (Verbrugge & Sevak, 2002). These feelings are fundamental to independence.

Among the most innovative new developments are a system that reminds a cognitively impaired person about the activities of daily living, a robotic assistant for impaired older persons at home, and electronic systems that provide cues to take medications. However, to have a meaningful impact on the lives of impaired older persons, efforts must be taken to assure that new technologies are accessible to the broad population of those in need.

THE DECISION TO MOVE

People prefer to stay in their homes and do so until their impairments severely affect their abilities to function and remain independent. The restrictions placed on housing adaptations and housing assistance may push many frail elderly to move to another, often more restrictive, environment. Moving is the last choice for most elderly, even those who may be considered frail.

The motivating factors to move are generally impairments in the instrumental activities of daily living (IADLs) such as shopping, cleaning, routine household chores, and cooking; and the absence of either a spouse or close relative to assist them (Longino, Jacobson, Zimmerman, & Bradsher, 1991; Reschovsky & Newman, 1990). Older adults often expect to move closer to an adult child out of need, particularly when they live alone and their health is poor (Silverstein & Angelelli, 1998). Informal supports play a dominant role in the ability of these elderly to remain in the community. Thus, the motivation to move is heightened when the individual is impaired and alone.

It is important to also note that assistance, even from informal supports, is more readily available for the sporadic tasks associated with home maintenance and home repair than for the daily assistance essential for maintaining independence. The frail elderly are more likely to find someone to fix a roof than to do cooking or laundry. But it is the absence of assistance with these routine tasks that can be the major influence on the decision to move.

It is not surprising that in a comparison of housing preferences and satisfaction between well and impaired elderly, the impaired were more dissatisfied with the amount of physical labor the house required (Gonyea, Hudson, & Seltzer, 1990). Moreover, those who were socially isolated from friends and family were more likely to anticipate a future move, although their strong preference was to remain in their homes with paid help for household and personal care.

Differences in the impetus to move exist between home owners and renters. Frail elderly who rent are more likely than frail home owners to move when their household needs exceed their capacity. Nevertheless, renters also prefer to remain in their established homes. By introducing supports they are frequently able to do so. Many of these supports appear to develop naturally through formal relationships.

In a survey of housing managers in San Francisco, Barker, Mitteness, and Wood (1988) found that landlords and managers of rental housing offered a wide variety of both formal and informal services to frail elderly long-term tenants, enabling them to remain in their apartments. Such assistance included grocery shopping, errands, housekeeping chores, and transportation.

Beyond the practical assistance that landlords and managers may offer to their frail tenants, there is also evidence that they are relied upon as important social supports. In a study of apartment managers of HUD-subsidized buildings in San Francisco, the managers were relied upon for help in a medical emergency. Moreover, the relationships between the elderly and these managers were strongly personalized, with managers describing the relationship as one of trust and dependability (Wolfson, Barker, & Mitteness, 1990). These same housing managers were better able to deal with physical than mental impairments among the tenants. They found it difficult to cope with confusion and behaviors that might be disruptive and even harmful to the tenant or others. Thus, these individuals were more likely to be evicted than those requiring only physical assistance or special housing adaptations.

RETIREMENT HOUSING

Retirement housing includes many types of planned residential programs. There is a wide range of such developments, from buildings that accept only residents over the age of 55 or 60, to facilities with services that help to maintain independence. The following discussion focuses on the latter type of facilities.

Naturally Occurring Retirement Communities

Naturally occurring retirement communities (NORCs) are apartment houses, complexes, or even neighborhoods in which a majority of the persons are over the age of 65. They develop because the residents in these areas have grown old there and want to remain. Services such as health care, counseling, social work, health education, and care management are generally provided to residents. Programs and services focus on assisting the residents to remain independent in their homes. More than 5,000 NORCs exist across the country, each offering a variety of programs. Findings from a national study on the role of NORCs indicate that they increase service availability to residents, provide services more cost-efficiently, and help in developing new resources for residents (Callahan & Lanspery, 1997).

The important role that NORCs can play in assisting older persons to remain in the community is reflected in the federal government's funding of five one-year demonstration programs in 2002, with funding given for the development of further programs in 2003. With the assistance of supportive services, the goal of these programs is to further enable older persons to age in place.

Continuing Care Retirement Communities

Continuing care retirement communities (CCRCs), or life care communities, integrate independent housing, assisted living, and nursing home care. They offer the feature of adjusting the environment to the needs of the older person. The communities typically provide personal care, social and recreational services, and congregate meals. The continuum of on-site services related to the changing functional status of the older person mean that residents are not at risk of eviction if they become impaired or their impairment worsens. Access to medical and long-term care services are often cited as reasons for moving into the communities.

A study of persons moving into a CCRC found the primary reasons for the move were the anticipation of future needs, a desire for care, freedom from maintaining a residence, and the desire not to be a burden on anyone (Krout et al., 2002). Further research on the satisfaction of residents indicates that women were more likely to be satisfied with the CCRC than men, while lower incomes and not wanting to live in a same-age community lowered satisfaction (Moen & Erikson, 2001).

The communities are geared toward the middle- and upper-income older population. Entrance fees typically range from $20,000 to more than $500,000, and monthly fees range from $600 to $3,200 depending on the areas, type of building, services provided, and the amount of health care needed. Many facilities require residents to sign contracts, and others offer rental units with specific fees for services. Generally there are three different types of fee schedules, one offering unlimited nursing care, one offering a base amount of care with the resident responsible for payments for more care, and those charging fees for service nursing care.

Thirty-eight states regulate CCRCs although there are no federal regulations. The Community Care Accreditation Commission of the American Association of Homes and Services for the Aging provides standards for the communities as well as accreditation. However, there is no requirement that programs and services participate in the commission. Consequently, older persons and their families contemplating a move to a CCRC need to be informed about the services provided and the extent to which it will meet their present and future needs. Because the programs offer health and supportive services as part of the contracts, they provide protection against many of the risks associated with aging and can offer many a sense of greater security.

Assisted Living

Assisted living facilities have continued to expand throughout the country as an alternative to nursing homes. There are approximately 33,000 assisted living facilities in the country serving more than 800,000 residents. Although they can serve very impaired people, in contrast to nursing homes the care is provided in more homelike settings, usually with persons having their own or a shared apartment. The goal of assisted living is to assure residents of choice, dignity, independence, autonomy, and a quality of life in their older years.

Services are supposed to be provided according to the level of need. Data from the National Center for Assisted Living (2001) show that the average resident needs help with 2.25 ADLs with only a minority, 19%, needing no help. These data also indicate that the typical resident is an 80-year-old woman requiring assistance with approximately 2 activities of daily living. Almost half of the residents move into assisted living from their own homes, while the majority leave because they require more extensive care.

Costs of the facilities vary greatly by region with the average monthly fee in 2000 being $1,873. Expected services include personal care, health care, social services, supervision when necessary, social and religious activities, recreation, transportation, and linen and housekeeping. However, as noted by in the first national survey on assisted living (Hawes, Rose, & Phillips, 1999), facilities differ greatly with regard to privacy and services offered. The cost of over 90% of assisted living is privately paid (American Health Care Association, 1998).

Most provide residents with a single room, with the remainder offering apartments for single occupancy. Although the majority admit residents with moderate physical limitations, fewer than half would admit persons requiring assistance moving from a bed or chair, or admit or retain persons with moderate or severe cognitive impairment. The survey found 65% of the facilities did not have a registered nurse on staff or provide nursing care, although they did offer 24-hour staff oversight, housekeeping, two meals a day, and personal assistance.

There are many areas of concern regarding assisted living that must be addressed before it can play a clear and substantial role in meeting the needs of the impaired older population. There is no clear definition of assisted living and no guidelines that distinguish it from other types of care facilities (Lewin-VHI, Inc. 1996). Lacking federal oversight or regulations, facilities vary in the services they offer and the types of residents they serve. Clarifying their role vis-á-vis that of nursing homes remains a key policy issue for states, particularly as states are increasingly using Medicaid to cover services in assisted living. In addition, with the majority of assisted living facilities privately owned, with more real estate developers and hotel managers than care providers (Stone, 2000), the motives of the industry itself have been questioned along with the amount of assistance actually provided.

Given the growth in assisted living and its potential role in the long-term care system, the Senate Committee on Aging held hearings with the intended outcome of ensuring the quality of the facilities. They wished to develop a foundation for policy and practices at both the federal and state levels. The final report issued in April 2003 (U.S. Senate Committee on Aging) outlined 110 recommendations for state and federal policy regarding the core principles of assisted living. Among these are recommendations to improve oversight of care, services, medication management, resident rights, and staffing. The report also recommends more regulation at the state level, making programs more accessible to lower-income and Medicaid-eligible persons, developing a national center for excellence, providing technical assistance to states, and developing outcome measures for residents.

Board and Care Homes

Board and care homes, also called residential care homes, personal care homes, domiciliary care homes, and homes for the aged, are similar to assisted living facilities in that they provide the same types of care, serving persons who have difficulty living independently. However, they concentrate on those with much lower incomes than does assisted living. Whereas assisted living developments, owned by large corporations, target upper-middle class persons, board and care homes are generally privately owned by lower income women in low-income communities and serve low-income older adults (Herd, 2001; Morgan, Eckert, & Lyon, 1995). Persons either have their own rooms or share one with another resident. Facilities are generally large homes or small apartment buildings. Many are in former hotels (Lewin-VHI, Inc. 1996).

Supplemental Security Income (SSI) finances the majority of persons living in board and care homes with many states providing supplements to the SSI payments. States may also pay for board and care through Medicaid funds or the Medicaid waiver. The cost of care in the homes is usually between 76% and 100% of the poverty-line income, with reimbursements to providers usually between $500 and $800 a month (Herd, 2001).

Persons moving into board and care homes generally lack any other options if they desire to remain in the community. Unfortunately, as with assisted living, board and care homes do not have any regulatory body certifying quality or standards. Moreover, one study (Morgan, Eckert, & Lyon, 1995) found 41% of board and care owners to be operating at a loss due to low SSI payments. Such low budgets impact on care as reflected in research showing a positive correlation between quality and cost (Lyon, 1997; Reschovsky & Ruchlin, 1993).

Board and care homes may be either licensed or unlicensed with regulations varying among the states. The Keys Amendments, enacted in 1976 as amendments to the Social Security Act, require states to identify group homes in which the majority of residents receive SSI, and to ensure that appropriate standards of care are set. The effectiveness of the amendments, however, has been seriously compromised in that they do not penalize substandard homes. Instead, the SSI payment to the resident is reduced. Furthermore, these requirements do not apply to unlicensed homes or those not serving SSI recipients.

A survey of facilities in states with different regulation requirements found that regulation does appear to be related to quality (Wildfire et al., 1998). Among the quality measures associated with licensure and regulation are safety, operators trained in care of the elderly, more supportive services, more recreational aids, greater staff knowledge of the aging process, and more assistive devices such as grab bars and raised toilet seats. In addition, states with stricter regulatory systems had fewer unlicensed facilities. Particularly important with regard to the needs of the frail elderly, board and care homes in states with limited regulations gave more psychotropic medications to the residents and were more likely to give medications contraindicated for the elderly. Otherwise, there was little difference with regard to regulation in meeting health care needs or in residents' rights.

Board and care homes can provide an important alternative to institutionalization for the impaired elderly; they occupy an important place in the continuum of housing options. The smaller settings and the greater informality of the residences can address many of these older individuals' needs for support. However, assuring the quality of these facilities is essential if they are to truly satisfy the requirements of this population.

FEDERALLY SPONSORED PROGRAMS

Federal housing designed specifically for elderly with service needs was first established in 1959 under the Section 202 Supportive Housing for the Elderly Program of the Department of Housing and Urban Development (HUD). The program continues to be the primary source of federal housing support for frail older persons. Section 202 provides capital for the development and expansion of supportive housing for low-income elderly, and offers rent subsidies for the residents to help cover the difference between the operating costs of the building and their individual rents. Rents are limited to 20% of the tenant's income. Since 1959, more than 5,000 housing projects with more than 260,000 units have been developed (Government Accounting Office (GAO), 1997).

Section 202 is intended to also ensure that residents have access to services that assist them to live independently, such as meals, transportation, personal assistance, and housekeeping. Housing managers are expected to be able to assess resident needs, coordinate services, and seek needed assistance. HUD provides some funding to projects that help with hiring service coordinators that link tenants with services.

Residents must be at least 62 years of age with an income below 50% of the area median income. Although the program has been extremely successful, units are in short supply, with long waiting lists. Additionally, turnover in the buildings is extremely low, with few persons choosing to move. In fact, the success of the buildings is attested to by the fact that transfers to a nursing home, or death, are the primary causes of vacancies.

A 1999 national survey of Section 202 housing found that approximately one third of all facilities surveyed had service coordinators on staff, while 43% reported that tenants had access to community service coordination (Heumann, Winter-Nelson, & Anderson, 2001). Those with staff coordinators reported that this was extremely positive for the developments and that it increased the range of services, enhanced quality, and permitted the residents to stay independent longer. Older facilities that tended to be larger, have more persons over the age of 80, more frail residents, and more persons able to pay privately for services, were the most likely to provide support services.

The capacity of Section 202 housing to stay current with the needs of the aging population is questionable. A survey by the Government Accounting Office (GAO, 2003) found serious delays in the construction of new units due to insufficient capital advances from HUD and an extremely slow process of approvals. The result is that housing is available to only 8% of very low-income elderly households (GAO, 2003). Funds for the development of 202 housing have continued to decline. At the same time, the extent to which these units and their services meet the needs of the residents or enable them to remain longer in the community is not clear.

Section 8 Housing

Section 8 provides rental assistance to low-income families, elderly, and disabled persons. A person is eligible for Section 8 if their gross income does not exceed 50% of HUD's median income guidelines. The program operates by providing vouchers to public housing authorities, to be used for partial payment of the rents of low-income persons. Similar to the Section 202 payments, these payments, made directly to the landlords, are usually the difference between the local standard payment and 30% of the tenants' income. To be part of the voucher program, the housing authority must show that it is responsive to the housing assistance needs of the tenants.

Participants in the program are free to choose any housing that accepts the voucher, signs an agreement with the housing authority, and of which the housing authority approves. However, there is a lack of clarity regarding the definition of "housing assistance needs." It is estimated that there were 2,100,000 vouchers issued in 2003, but the long waiting lists of 2 to 10 years for this housing suggests that these do not meet the need—although no new vouchers are being offered. In addition, many contracts with housing facilities are expiring and not being renewed, leading to a further shortage of units. Consequently, many older persons have been either displaced from housing or are unable to find housing. There is a further concern about efforts to place the voucher program into block grants to the states, a plan that would result in varying regulations and priorities, and certainly place the older population in competition for housing with other groups.

Congregate Housing Services Program

In order to meet the support needs of the frail elderly in these subsidized units, the Congregate Housing Services Program (CHSP), the only part of HUD to provide social services, was initiated in 1978. The program was designed to serve all residents eligible for Section 202 housing identified as vulnerable by local assessment committees (LACs). The goal was to prevent these individuals from having to enter institutions. CHSP provides service coordination, housekeeping, personal care, congregate meals, and transportation to frail elderly and younger persons with disabilities. Its intent is to maximize this population's independence, assisting management in meeting their needs, and ensuring that needed services are available.

The CHSP offers grants to states, local government, public housing authorities, and nonprofit organizations to provide meals and other services to elderly and disabled tenants of federally supported housing. HUD pays for 40% of the costs of services, the grantees are responsible for 50%, and the residents must pay at least 10% of the costs. The primary service offered to tenants is meals, with HUD requiring that 2 meals a day, 7 days a week be provided. Nonmedical services offered through the CHSP include housekeeping, personal assistance, transportation, escort, and social services. Fees are based on the older individual's ability to pay. Although funds have been allocated to maintain existing programs, however, no new programs have been funded since 1995.

Hope for Elderly Independence Demonstration Program

The Hope for Elderly Independence Demonstration Program (HOPE IV), administered by HUD, was funded in 1993 for 5 years as another model for providing assistance to the frail elderly to help maintain them in the community. It provided grants for supportive services and rental assistance to frail older persons in Section 8 rental housing. The program focused on developing services for low-income elderly persons (62 and older) with limitations in three or more ADLs. In order to receive services, persons had to be assessed by a service coordinator who then developed a care plan and arranged for assistance. In contrast to CHSP, which develops services in public housing, HOPE IV is based on the needs of individual tenants who do not have to live in one facility. Unlike CHSP, the program serves only the frail elderly and not the younger disabled.

An evaluation of Project Hope (Ficke & Berkowitz, 2000) found that participants, despite their increasing frailty, reported that they were satisfied with their lives, liked their neighborhoods and living arrangements, were confident and had few worries, had good appetites, and felt in control of their lives. The evaluators concluded that even the frailest elderly who are also low-income and have few or no support systems are able to live independently in a service-rich environment that includes case management.

A comparison of the effectiveness of CHSP and HOPE IV found that both were important in meeting the needs of the frail elderly in the community and that each created partnerships with service delivery systems (Ficke, Berkowitz, & Westate, 2000). Among the reports recommendations are the following:

1) Expand service coordinator programs of congregate housing into HUD tenant-based programs.
2) Increase the adoption of CHSP and HOPE models for HUD tenants and residents, as well as for the new Section 8 voucher and congregate housing applicants as a means of meeting the high level of needs of the elderly.
3) Ensure that frail seniors have a range of housing assistance options rather than attempting to meet them in the scattered sites of housing projects.

Low-Income Housing Tax Credits

The Low-Income Housing Tax Credit program (LIHTC) is the primary federal subsidy program for the development of rental housing for lower income persons. At least 20%–40% of units must serve low-income residents. LIHTC develops more units annually, 15,000, than the 10,000 created by Section 202 housing. Tax credits are given by states to specific developers who then either renovate older buildings or construct new housing. One of the criteria used by states in providing the credits is that the housing will serve a specific population with special needs. The elderly constitute one of these special-needs groups though they may also live in projects that serve diverse age groups. Most developments are in rural or suburban areas with very few in central cities where the majority of low-income elderly reside. Section 8 vouchers can be used in LIHTC housing.

A survey of these units show that approximately one quarter were developed specifically for older persons and that this group is more likely to have impairments than those living in mixed-age facilities (Kochera, 2002). Approximately one third of those living in LIHTC housing specifically for the elderly had some type of impairment in their ADL functioning.

The survey found waiting lists of approximately 8 months for almost all units for older persons. These units were more likely to have accessibility features such as grab bars in bathrooms and outside ramps than did mixed resident buildings. Unlike Section 202 housing, the LIHTC program does not include a service coordinator. However, nearly half of the programs for older adults had access to a service coordinator and offered services, primarily social and recreational programs. As the program does not provide a subsidy for supportive services, these are obtained through state funding, Medicaid, or other organizations.

The findings suggest that LIHTC may be an important means for the federal government to develop housing for the impaired low-income older population. An analysis made by HUD of allocations for 2002 found that 88% of states used their funds for developments primarily for the elderly (HUD, 2003). Concerns about the ability of the program to expand to meet the needs of the older population continue since the program depends greatly on the willingness and ability of private developers to invest.

OTHER HOUSING OPTIONS

Shared Housing

Shared housing programs offer a potential means for frail elderly to remain in their own homes. The programs involve sharing an existing house with at least one other person in exchange for either rent or services or both. Shared housing can therefore be particularly important in meeting the needs of the older home owner with some functional impairment. The National Shared Housing Resource Center offers technical assistance for the development of shared housing programs, as well was as a directory of shared housing programs throughout the United States.

A study of homesharing participants in Wisconsin found that the functional status of the home provider set up the framework for understanding the type of assistance they required and the kind and amount of resources to be exchanged (Jaffe & Howe, 1989). Healthy elderly home owners were interested in having someone in the house at night and assistance with some home maintenance in exchange for reduced rent. A second group of elderly were those with some functional limitations who needed assistance with basic household tasks such as cooking and shopping. These home owners were willing to offer free room and board in exchange for these services. The third group were those who were so physically or mentally frail that they required almost constant supervision. This group offered free room and board in exchange for this supervision, and also a small stipend for services.

A study of homesharing in one of the oldest programs, Operation Match, in San Jose, California, detailed the primary reasons for sharing given by both providers and seekers as financial need and companionship (Pynoos, Hamburger, & June, 1990). Elderly providers were most likely to share because of a need for help or security, rather than companionship. Meal preparation, housework, and laundry were the tasks commonly required by the home owner. Assistance with heavier chores was generally not given. Contrary to the findings discussed above, levels of dependency were not necessarily correlated with assistance and services were not necessarily rendered by the sharer.

Homesharing enables many elderly to exchange an important resource, the home, for needed services. The program can impact on both the instrumental and affective states of the older person. It can offer real assistance and support in the home while also strengthening the sense of control of the older person, because he or she holds something of value which can be exchanged for services (Danigelis & Fengler, 1990). Homesharing can also reduce the demands for care placed on the family and on formal services.

There are varying types of homesharing programs. In its simplest form, an agency, often a office within the local department of aging, acts as an intermediary between the home owner and the would-be sharer, screening the two to determine compatibility. Once the arrangement between the two is made, the agency has no further role. In other programs, the agency continues in a case management role to assist with the relationship. This case management role is particularly important when the home owners seeking to share are extremely frail and dependent. In these instances, the homeseeker is expected to provide needed assistance to the owner. These expectations and requirements may not always be clear and thus the intervention by a case manager is warranted.

In a study of the case management function in shared housing, Jaffe and Howe (1989) found that it is relatively unnecessary when the home owner is well and independent. For elderly in a more transitional state, requiring some assistance from the sharer, case management can play a meaningful role. In situations in which the home owner is dependent due to mental or physical impairments and the person sharing is expected to provide care, case management is most important and needs to play an active role in the relationship.

With correct management and agency involvement, shared housing offers a responsive option in meeting the needs of the older population. By offering financial assistance as well as services, social interaction, and a renewed sense of self-worth, the program can enable many with varying functional impairments to continue to live in their own homes.

ECHO Housing

ECHO, or "elder cottage housing opportunity" began in the United States in the late 1970s but has had limited popularity due to zoning restrictions and the cautious involvement of both government and potential consumers. Originally known as "granny flats," the program is modeled after one originating in Australia (Folts & Muir, 2002).

ECHO housing consists of special units constructed for the elderly, usually on the property of relatives. They offer the elderly independence but close proximity to those who can offer support and assistance. The units are usually temporary and thus can be removed when no longer needed.

Several benefits may make ECHO housing most attractive to the elderly (Hare, 1991). The housing fosters independence by having the elderly in easy access to support systems but not completely dependent on them. The housing is also low-cost and can assist the elderly to obtain needed funds. By selling larger homes and moving into less expensive ECHO housing, elderly home owners can realize profits that can be used to meet living expenses.

Barriers to this type of housing exist in many localities, particularly with regard to zoning. Zoning restrictions that require long waits for approval can significantly deter many elderly who need to move quickly due to deteriorating environmental or health conditions. Zoning in many localities prohibits multiple dwellings on any tract of land, although amendments can be made for individual cases in which the resident applies for a permit to care for an elderly parent (Hare, 1991, op cit.). However, these types of restrictions can impede the development of this type of housing because many families lack the motivation to challenge such regulations. Moreover, by the time regulations are met, the housing may no longer be appropriate for the relative.

Adult Foster Care

Adult foster care is another option for assisting functionally impaired older persons to remain in the community. As with foster care programs for children, most homes are operated by private families and provide care for a small number of adults. Room and board, assistance with activities of daily living, and supervision are provided.

Licensing of adult foster care homes varies, with some states having no licensing provisions. Consequently, the number of persons in the home as well as provided services also vary. Payments are usually made by the older person with the assistance of some subsidies, while services may be covered under Medicaid waivers or other state programs.

A study of adult foster care in Oregon found that its costs were less than that of nursing homes (Kane, Ilston, Kane, & Nyman, 1990). Moreover, foster care residents were less disabled than nursing home residents; Medicaid residents were less disabled than private-pay residents. Residents chose foster care for its flexibility, while nursing home residents selected homes for their organized activities and rehabilitation opportunities.

SUMMARY

Most older persons desire to remain in their own homes as long as possible. The ability of these individuals to do so is often restricted by a lack of housing options or alternatives. Programs, services, and even technological devices that can enable them to remain in their homes are often not available or accessible to those in need.

Without adequate resources many elderly are forced to move to more restricted environments or even nursing homes in order to receive needed support and assistance. As the chapter has discussed, independence-promoting alternatives are available, including home modifications and technological devices, but their availability tends toward those who can afford them. For many, access to such programs is beyond their economic means.

The government has become increasingly aware of the needs of older persons wishing to remain in the community. It has become cognizant of the impact support services can have to prevent institutionalization, through programs such as Section 202 housing. However, though sensitive policies and programs have been established, they remain fragmented, in jeopardy, or have been discontinued. For other programs, such as Section 8 housing, their effectiveness and impact in meeting the needs of older persons is diminished due to inadequate funding and long waiting lists. Moreover, proposals to block-grant the program may further jeopardize its role in meeting the needs of older persons, as they are placed in competition with other populations who do not share the same service needs.

The many types of housing programs that exist can provide a real continuum of options for independent living. Assisted living, which continues to expand throughout the country, is an example of a program that can promote autonomy and independence. However, with regulations and standards lacking and with most facilities beyond the means of those with the greatest needs, the role of these programs in serving the vast population of impaired older persons is questionable. By assuring that they provide effective and appropriate services and that these are affordable to a greater proportion of older persons, either by accepting public funding such as Medicaid or SSI payments, or reducing fees, they could assume an important role in the care continuum.

As the older population continues to represent diverse backgrounds and needs, a plethora of housing options is essential. Most fundamental to the housing needs of this population are programs and services that can assist them to remain as long as possible, with dignity, in their own homes. In the long run, such programs can be far more cost effective than building more housing or moving individuals to more sheltered environments.

REFERENCES

American Health Care Association (AHCA). (1998). *Facts and trends: The assisted living sourcebook.* Washington, DC: National Center for Assisted Living.

Barker, J. C., Mitteness, L. S., & Wood, S. J. (1988). Gatekeeping: Residential managers and elderly tenants. *Gerontologist, 28,* 625–631.

Callahan, J., & Lanspery, S. (1997, January–March). Can we tap the power of NORCs? In *Perspective on aging.* Grants Results Report. Washington, DC: National Council on Aging.

Christenson, M. (1990). *Aging in the designed environment.* New York: Haworth Press.

Coordinated Care Management Corporation. (1989). *Personal emergency response system demonstration project.* Buffalo, NY: Author.

Danigelis, N., & Fengler, A. (1990). Homesharing: How social exchange helps elders live at home. *Gerontologist, 30,* 162–170.

Ficke, R., & Berkowitz, S. (1999). *Evaluation of the HOPE for elderly independence demonstration, Final Report.* Rockville, MD: Westat Inc.

Ficke, R., Berkowitz, S., & Westate (2000). *Evaluation of the hope for elderly independence demonstration program and the new congregate housing services program: Report to congress.* U.S. Department of Housing and Urban Development. Rockville, MD: Westat Inc.

Folts, W., & Muir, K. (2002). Housing for older adults: New lessons from the past. *Research on Aging, 24,* 10–28.

Gaberlavage, G., & Forsythe, P. (1995). *Home repair and modification; A survey of city programs.* Washington, DC: American Association of Retired Persons, Public Policy Institute.

Gonyea, J., Hudson, R., & Seltzer, G. (1990). Housing preferences of vulnerable elders in suburbia. *Journal of Housing for the Elderly, 1*(2), 79–95.

Government Accounting Office (GAO). (2003). *Project funding and other factors that delay assistance to needy households,* GAO-03-512. Washington, DC: Government Printing Office.

Hare, P. (1991). The ECHO housing/granny flat experience in the U.S. *Journal of Housing for the Elderly, 7,* 57–70.

Hawes, C., Rose, M., & Phillips, C. (1999). *A national study of assisted living for the frail elderly. Executive summary: Results of a national survey of facilities.* Beachwood, OH: Mewers Research Institute.

Herd, P. (2001). Vertical axes on the long-term care continuum: A comparison of board and care and assisted living. *Journal of Aging and Social Policy, 13,* 37–56.

Heumann, L., Winter-Nelson, K., & Anderson, J. (2001). *1999 national survey of Section 202 elderly housing.* (No. 2001-02). Washington, DC: Public Policy Institute, American Association of Retired Persons.

Housing and Urban Development. (2003). *Analysis of state qualified allocation plans for the low income housing tax credit.* Washington, DC: U.S. Department of Housing and Urban Development.

Jaffe, D., & Howe, E. (1989). Case management for homesharing. *Journal of Gerontological Social Work, 14,* 91–110.

Kane, R., Ilston, L., Kane, L., & Nyman, J. (1990). *Meshing services with housing: Lessons from adult foster care and assisted living in Oregon.* Minneapolis, MN: Division of Health Services Research and Policy.

Kochera, N. (2002). *Serving the affordable housing needs of older low-income renters: A survey of low-income housing tax credit properties.* Washington, DC: AARP, Public Policy Institute.

Krout, J., Moen, P., Holmes, H., Oggins, J., & Bowen, N. (2002). Reasons for relocation to a continuing care retirement community. *Journal of Applied Gerontology, 21,* 236–256.

Lewin-VHI, Inc. (1996). *National study of assisted living for the frail elderly. Literature review update.* Contract No. HHS-1-94-0024. Fairfax, VA: Author:

Longino, C., Jackson, D., Zimmerman, R., & Bradsher, J. (1991). The second move: Health and geographic mobility. *Journal of Gerontology, 46,* S218–S225.

Louie, J. (1999). *Housing modifications for disabled elderly households.* Joint Center for Housing Studies, Graduate School of Design and John F. Kennedy School of Government. Cambridge, MA: Harvard University.

Lyon, S. (1997). Impact of regulation and financing on small board and cares in Maryland. *Journal of Aging and Social Policy, 9,* 37–50.

Mann, W. (1997). Common telecommunications technology for promoting safety, independence, and social interaction for older people with disabilities. *Generations, 21,* 18–19.

Mathieson, K., Kronefeld, J., & Keith, V. (2002). Maintaining functional independence in elderly adults: The roles of health status and financial resources in predicting home modifications and use of mobility equipment. *Gerontologist, 42,* 24–31.

Moen, P., & Erikson, M. (2001). Decision making and satisfaction with a continuing care retirement community. *Journal of Housing for the Elderly, 14,* 53–69.

Morgan, L., Eckert, J., & Lyon, S. (1995). *Board and care homes: Residential care in transition.* Baltimore, MD: Johns Hopkins University Press.

National Center for Assisted Living. (2001). *2000 survey of assisted living facilities.* Washington, DC: American Health Care Association.

Newman, S. (2003). The living conditions of elderly Americans. *Gerontologist, 43,* 99–109.

Pynoos, J. (1993). Toward a national policy on home modification. *Technology and Disability, 2,* 1–8.

Pynoos, J. (1992). Strategies for home modification and repair. *Generations, 16,* 21–25.

Pynoos, J., Hamburger, L., & June, A. (1990). Supportive relationships in shared housing. *Journal of Housing for the Elderly, 6,* 1–24.

Reschovsky, J., & Newman, S. (1990). Adaptations for independent living by older frail households. *Gerontologist, 30,* 543–552.

Reschovsky, J., & Ruchlin, H. (1993). Quality of board and care homes serving the low-income elderly: Structural and public policy correlates. *Journal of Applied Gerontology, 12,* 225–245.

Silverstein, M., & Angelelli, J. (1998). Older persons' expectations of moving closer to their children. *Journal of Gerontology, Series B, Psychological Sciences and Social Sciences, 53B,* S153–S163.

Stone, R. (2000). *Long-term care for the elderly with disabilities: Current policy, emerging trends, and implications for the twenty-first century.* New York: Milbank Memorial Fund.

Struyk, R., & Katsura, H. (1988). *Aging at home: How the elderly adjust their housing without moving.* New York: Haworth Press.

U.S. Senate Committee on Aging. (2003). *Assisted living workgroup final report, special committee on aging.* Washington, DC: U.S. Government Printing Office.

Verbrugge, L., & Sevak, P. (2002). Use, type, and efficacy as assistance for disability. *Journal of Gerontology, Psychological Sciences and Social Sciences, 57,* 366–379.

Wildfire, J., Hawes, C., More, V., Lux, L., & Brown, F. (1998). Effect of regulation on the quality of care in board and care homes. *Generations, 21,* 25–29.

Wolfson, C., Barker, J., & Mitteness, L. (1990). Personalization of formal social relationships by the elderly. *Research on Aging, 12*(1), 94–112.

The Role of the Family in Providing Care

Chronic impairments affecting functioning become more common as persons age, and so do does their need for assistance, particularly if they are to remain in the community. The bulwark of this assistance is provided by the family, with family members providing 60%–80% of the long-term care for dependent relatives (Bengston, Rosenthal, & Burton, 1996). Estimates show that disabled older persons receive approximately 120 million hours of informal assistance each year, with the majority provided by family members. The economic value of this care is estimated at between $45 billion and $94 billion per year (Stone, 2000). Being married reduced the risk of entering a nursing home by 41%, having at least one daughter reduced risk by 27%, and having at least one living sibling reduced it by 21% (Freedman, 1996).

THE CAREGIVING RELATIONSHIP

Reciprocity is often given as a motive for helping and providing care to an older adult. According to the norm of reciprocity, people feel obligated to assist those who have cared for them at various points in their lives. To not reciprocate such care is to recant on a normative responsibility. Reciprocity provides a basis for social relationships in that each person in the dyad is expected to both give and receive assistance. In caring for an older relative, the spouse and children are the ones most likely to be bound by this norm. However, many, more distant relatives, and even friends, may perceive their caregiving activities as a means of repaying a longstanding debt to the frail individual.

Family and friends are also motivated to aid the frail by feelings of commitment and ties of affection. These sentiments appear to underlie many helping relationships and to remain strong without regard to distance or social class (Litwak, 1985). In fact, the affection transmitted through the relationship may be important to the well-being of the older person by reinforcing their social involvement (Antonnucci & Depner, 1982).

However, the demands engendered in the caregiving relationship can also have negative effects on both caregiver and receiver. A failure to respond to the needs of the frail individual can result in feelings of guilt in many family members. These feelings, and the need to compensate for them, may influence caregivers' involvement. In those instances where there is no improvement in the condition of the frail relative, regardless of the amount of assistance, the guilt can be hard to overcome.

Research (Pruchno, Burant, & Peters, 1997) has also examined the impact of caregiving on the care receiver and the dyadic relationship between giver and receiver. The level of stress experienced by the caregiver is influenced by his or her assessment of the situation. At the same time, as the care receiver feels able to contribute to the family, his or her sense of control and psychological well-being are enhanced. Being able to give as well as receive can thus empower both care receiver and caregiver and strengthen the relationship.

Further research on the dyadic relationship between caregivers and care receivers indicates that caregivers are likely to perceive the care recipients as more dependent than the recipients perceive themselves (Lyons, Zarit, Sayer, & Whitlatch, 2002). In addition, as caregivers experienced more strain in the caregiving relationship, they experienced greater caregiver difficulties. These difficulties were not perceived by the care recipient, suggesting that disagreements regarding the situation and needs can be a source of stress to each member.

Specific cultural norms can greatly influence the caring relationship. Values of filial piety that emphasize respect for elders and the responsibility of the family to provide care to elderly relatives remain strong among many ethnic groups. Relatives who do not adhere to such behaviors are in danger of being treated as deviants within their immediate cultural groups. Moreover, to the extent that they themselves maintain these traditional values, they are susceptible to feeling guilty for not completely fulfilling them.

Frail elderly who continue to both expect and demand assistance from their children and other relatives frequently reinforce these normative behaviors. For these families, using any type of formal service may be interpreted as failing to fulfill one's responsibilities. This is why, in attempting to understand caregiving activities, it is essential to examine the ethnic characteristics of the elderly and their caregivers.

THEORETICAL PERSPECTIVES

Theoretical perspectives provide a context for caregiving relationships to be understood while also permitting some prediction of the outcome of the relationship. Such perspectives establish a basis for designing interventions that may strengthen the relationship and better assure that it meets the needs of both the caregiver and care receiver.

Social Exchange

Exchange theory views all social interaction as an exchange between two actors in which each seeks to maximize rewards and minimize costs (Dowd, 1980). Individuals will continue in the exchange only as long as it is perceived as more rewarding than costly.

This theory views older persons as having diminished resources in relationships, as they possess little of value to others. As a means of protecting themselves from feelings of dependency, they may withdraw from social interactions. As discussed by Lee (1985), this lack of power in the exchange may account for findings suggesting that older persons receive more gratification in their relationships with friends than with relatives. The former are more likely to be based on mutual interests and rewards, while the latter may be more influenced by duty and obligation which intensify the feelings of dependency. Elderly who are unable to reciprocate in relationships with their children are likely to have a devalued sense of well-being and lower morale than those who are able to reciprocate (Stoller, 1985).

The complexity of the caregiving relationship with regard to social exchange is underscored by contrasting findings that imply that assistance from adult children can be associated with increased morale. In a study of elderly widows, Mutran and Reitzes (1984) found that higher morale was positively associated with receiving more assistance. The receipt of assistance was perceived as a reward and as making the exchange gratifying.

Concurrently, giving more in a relationship is not necessarily supportive of well-being. A study of exchange between elderly mothers and their adult daughters found that mothers' offering financial assistance as a means to feel less dependent and reduce the power imbalance in the relationship did not necessarily restructure the balance, as the mothers continued to feel devalued (Talbott, 1990). In fact, many complained that the children did not offer sufficient help and that they continued to feel a burden to them.

While some research has shown no relationship between receiving assistance and morale (Lee & Ellithorpe, 1982), other studies (Liang, Krause, & Bennett, 2001) indicate that both giving and receiving have positive and negative effects on well-being. Any lack of association may be due to the fact that these older persons have additional systems or exchange dimensions that are not being measured and are based on previous exchanges. In most cases, well-being is sustained even when the older person is dependent and receives assistance.

The conflicting results of these studies highlight the complexity involved in understanding the caregiving relationship and its effects on the frail older person. In some instances, there may be few effects. In others the receipt of assistance may be harmful to emotional well-being by fostering a sense of dependency, or it may reaffirm social ties and relationships. Consequently, the uniqueness of the relationship, the characteristics of both caregiver and older person, and their own personal histories must be considered when interpreting the effects on well-being of the frail individual.

Continuity Theory and Caregiving

From the perspective of continuity theory, dependency can be particularly demoralizing to the individual who was previously accustomed to being the authority figure. Accepting a new dependent role is tangible evidence that the former ways of behaving are no longer possible, making role continuity difficult to maintain. Accordingly, the most deleterious effects on morale may occur in those for whom dependency poses the sharpest contrast to previous roles and thus the most discontinuity.

At the same time, continuity theory assumes that all individuals seek to maintain roles to which they are accustomed and that they find rewarding. It may be anticipated that any discontinuity may be just as problematic for the caregiver. Thus, the spouse or adult child accustomed to being dependent on the now-frail older individual may find the role of caregiver difficult to accept. This altered dyadic relationship will require a major shift in behaviors, as traditional roles are no longer appropriate. On the other hand, to the extent that the caregiving role is a continuation of earlier patterns of interaction in that the frail individual was previously dependent, both spousal and child caregivers should have an easier time of accommodating the demands associated with the impairments.

Feminism and Caregiving

Feminist theory examines how cultures and societies create gender, the relations between gender, and the norms and roles associated with gender. Feminist gerontology examines how gender affects the aging process, roles, and position of older women. With gender socially created, the experiences encountered by older women are the result of social structure, social policies, and gender-based inequities. By understanding how gender and gender relations are created by a society, efforts can be made to alter the attitudes and norms that maintain such inequities. According to feminist theory, the dominance of women in caregiving is not the result of particular nurturing or emotional qualities, but rather a socialization process and policies that stem from a society's dependence on women's unpaid labor, which exhausts their roles as caregivers (Hooyman, 1999; Stoller, 1994).

Postmodern feminists examine the way language itself affects thought and reality (Ray, 1999). As language is socially constructed it defines relationships and can exaggerate and distort what is actually occurring. Ray provides the example of caregiver-care receiver distinction, that depicts an active care "giver" in relation to a passive care "receiver." The labels do not account for any efforts the receiver may be making on his or her own behalf. Postmodern feminists deconstruct "caregiving" to two assumptions: that "care" involves intimacy and connection and that the meeting of physical needs is offered freely ("given"). Thus, excluded from classification as caregiver would be those being paid for their assistance and those providing help out of a sense of duty and responsibility.

Feminist theory elucidates the way in which the social structure and its inequities contribute to woman's' role as caregiver to older persons, as well as to the stresses they may experience. Whereas an individualist approach would aim to improve the woman's adjustment to the role through therapy or support groups, a feminist perspective targets structural arrangements of work and caregiving that create women's dependency and low economic status in old age (Hooyman, 1999).

MODELS OF CAREGIVING

Models are used to describe relationships between variables and their outcomes. With regard to caregiving, these models suggest which factors may affect the well-being of both caregiver and care receiver. In general, these models have concentrated on the factors contributing to stress among caregivers. The stress of caregiving is viewed as resulting from competing roles, the caregiver's perceptions of the stressors, and caregiver resources in dealing with patient behaviors. Two broader models of the caregiving relationship that seek to explain both positive and negative interactions as well as effects on the care recipient are those offered by Young and Kahana (1989) and Roberts and Bengston (1990).

The model of caregiving presented by Young and Kahana (1989) views several patient and caregiver variables as influencing the outcome of the caregiving relationship. Attitudinal behavioral, sociodemographic, and health characteristics of caregiver and patient, as well as the extent of care and the home environment, contribute to the well-being of both. Hence gender, relationship, and living situation are important factors to consider when attempting to understand the outcome of a caregiving situation.

Roberts and Bengtson's (1990) model of intergenerational family relations posits familial norms regarding closeness, affection, intergenerational contacts, and the exchange of resources as being a basis for interaction and assistance. Within this framework, a balanced exchange of resources contributes to positive feelings and affection as well as more assistance.

In their empirical test of the model, helping behavior by adult children was a predictor of their affection and their ties with parents. Such behavior reflects the adult child's endorsement of norms of filial responsibility, the dependency needs of the older individual, and the proximity of the adult child to the parent. One can conclude that the stronger the feelings of affection, sense of filial responsibility, and ability to offer help, the greater should be the involvement. On the other hand, the theory also suggests that children who are not able to act on their feelings, such as those separated by distance, may be particularly susceptible to stress.

WHO ARE THE CAREGIVERS?

Data from the 1994 Disability Supplement to the National Long Term Care Survey provides the most complete description of informal caregivers of the elderly (Agency for Healthcare Research and Quality, 2001). In 1994, there were 5.9 million informal caregivers providing care for the 3.6 million elderly in the United States. The data show that 63% of these caregivers are women. Spouses compose approximately 23%

of the caregivers, and approximately 44% of the caregivers were adult children with daughters composing the majority (27%) of this group. Eighty-seven percent of the caregivers were White; Blacks accounted for 12%. One third of the caregivers cared for persons with three or more ADL limitations.

Given the needs of this population, it is important to note that almost half (40%) of these older persons depended only on informal assistance, with one quarter receiving both informal and formal care. About 30% of caregivers were themselves over the age of 65, with another 15% between the ages of 45 and 54.

Data from a national survey of family caregivers (National Alliance for Caregiving and American Association of Retired Persons, 1997) show that the average caregiver is a married, 46-year-old woman who is also employed outside the home. The survey also found that 20% of these caregivers care for someone with mental confusion, dementia, Alzheimer's disease, or forgetfulness.

A survey by the Metropolitan Life Insurance Company (1999) underscores the impact that caregiving has on employed caregivers. Two in 10 caregivers surveyed reported turning down work on special projects or travel-related work in order to provide care. Forty percent claimed that caregiving affected their ability to advance in their jobs. Caregivers also underestimated the duration of time that they would spend caregiving, with 46% estimating that it would be more than 2 years. However, the average length of caregiving was 8 years, with one third of the respondents caregiving for 10 years or more. Caregivers reported a loss of income since their caregiving lessened their opportunities for advancement, increased their absenteeism, and for many resulted in early retirement.

Studies of caregiving indicate a hierarchical pattern for care with older persons turning first to spouses, then to adult children, other relatives, and friends (Coward, Horne, & Dwyer, 1992). Proximity is also important in determining the caregiver, because adult children living close to the older person are likely to assume the role. In addition, studies have found that even when a secondary caregiver is available to provide assistance, the primary caregiver did not reduce or alter the type of assistance he or she offered (Penrod, Kane, Kane, & Finch, 1995).

The dependency needs of the frail, whether spouse or parent, alter established relationships and interactions, necessitating new patterns of behavior. Fundamental to this process is the acceptance by both the older person and the caregiver of the impairment and its ensuing limitations. In order to maintain the highest level of functioning of elderly, however, it is essential that the acknowledgement of needs for assistance not diminish their sense of self-esteem.

Spousal Caregivers

Data continue to indicate that spousal caregivers are more likely to be wives than husbands, as women, both wives and daughters, continue to be the most active caregivers (Spillman & Pezzin, 2000). Spousal caregivers face particular challenges, as they tend to be older than other caregivers and to often suffer from poor health themselves. Indeed, the act of caregiving can further affect their health as it increasingly encompasses their lives (Burton, Zdaniuk, Schulz, Jackson, & Hirsh, 2003).

As difficult as caregiving may be, however, there is some evidence to suggest that its effects are not uniformly deleterious. A spouse's reaction to caregiving appears to also be influenced by the nature of their relationship prior to the illness. Couples who had been mutually responsive to each other have been found to be less depressed as caregivers and more inclined to report their caregiving relationship as rewarding (Williamson & Shaffer, 2001). Having had a positive relationship before the illness is conducive to spouses feeling rewarded and effective as caregivers (Seltzer & Wailing Li, 1996). Studies have shown that spousal caregivers can gain satisfaction, a sense of worth, and increased self-esteem from the caregiving role, regardless of the level of burden they experience (Kramer, 1997; Seltzer & Wailing Li, 1996).

Gender also informs spousal caregiving. Older wives caring for an impaired husband may perceive this care as an extension of their usual role. Husbands providing care often begin to redefine their sense of worth separate from their work role (Kramer, 1997). In a large survey of women and men over age 70 living in the community, Katz (2000) found that disabled wives cared for by husbands receive fewer hours of informal assistance than husbands being cared for by wives. In addition, wives were the primary caregivers of older disabled men while women, mainly daughters, were the primary caregivers of older disabled women. In addition, research has noted that husbands experience spousal care as more problematic than do wives (Marks, Lambert, & Choi, 2002) although women, both wives and daughters, are more likely to report feeling strain as caregivers (National Alliance of Caregiving and American Association of Retired Persons, 1997).

Elderly spouses who report strain associated with their caregiving have an increased risk of themselves dying (Shulz & Beach, 1999).

Increases in mortality and morbidity may be linked to feelings of burden and strain, as they are at least partially associated with poorer health behaviors of the caregivers. Spouses reporting more burden, depression, and involvement in more caregiving tasks have also been found to consume more alcohol, exercise less, and smoke more than those feeling less burdened and depressed (Gallant & Connell, 1997).

Adult Children as Caregivers

Adult children, mostly daughters, are the primary caregivers of older adults. Although daughters are the primary caregivers, however, sons also participate. Sons' assistance tends to be less extensive, though (Horowitz, 1985; Wolf, Freedman, & Soldo, 1997). In addition, types of assistance provided vary by gender. Daughters are more likely to help with personal care such as bathing, dressing, and eating (Lee, Dwyer, & Coward, 1993). Men are more likely to help with transportation, finances, case management, and occasional household chores (Connadis, Rosenthal, & McMullin, 1996).

The likelihood of receiving any assistance from an adult child increases with the number of living children (Spitze & Logan, 1990), and having more children is positively associated with more hours of help (Soldo, Agree, & Wolf, 1989). However, studies have also found that with more children to provide assistance, any one child's involvement can be reduced (Wolf et al., 1997). Not all older parents receive such assistance. Divorce can negatively affect the involvement of adult children as caregivers, as their ties to the parent are weakened, with older fathers particularly vulnerable (Schone & Pezzin, 1999).

Although the major responsibility for caring for the frail elderly is assumed by adult daughters and daughters-in-law, this is not without some stress. At the time of life when they begin providing this care they are frequently meeting caregiving responsibilities in their own families or are anticipating a period of growth as their caregiving comes to an end. Instead, their own desires are frequently overshadowed by the dependency needs of parents or parents-in-law.

That women continue to accept the caregiving role has been attributed to feelings of reciprocity for past caregiving, affection, norms, and values. Whether wives or daughters, they have been socialized to be expressive, nurturing, and responsive to the needs of others, defining themselves according to relationships (Chodorow, 1978). These characteristic feminine traits make it difficult for women to ignore the needs of frail and dependent parents. Moreover, studies have also shown that older children continue to provide for their parents even when their own health is failing (Laditka & Laditka, 2000). Finally, studies have indicated that in comparison with male caregivers, women have more difficulty balancing their caregiving with other responsibilities and have poorer emotional health (Naivaie-Waliser, Spriggs, & Feldman, 2002).

Primary and Secondary Caregivers

Most older persons requiring assistance are not dependent on one person, but a network of helpers ranging between two and four (Stephens & Christenson, 1986; Stoller & Pugliesi, 1991). Primary caregivers are those who offer the majority of the care, frequently sharing the household with the older person. Secondary caregivers play important roles in the assistance they offer, with their work often coordinated by the primary caregiver. In many instances these secondary caregivers are children or the spouse of the primary caregiver and offer intermittent help such as shopping, transportation, and home repairs. Although important in the caregiving relationship, secondary caregivers will not necessarily substitute for the primary caregiver if that person is unable to continue in the role (Cox & Monk, 1990; Penrod, Kane, Kane, & Finch, 1995).

Among siblings, tension can develop when the principal caregiver feels that the other caregivers are not doing enough, especially as the needs for care increase (Brody, Hoffman, Kleban, & Schoonhover, 1989). The caregiving itself can result in stress among family members as the roles and involved tasks become more demanding. In some instances, this stress is compounded when the primary caregiver becomes absorbed in the role and finds it difficult to share tasks with others. Thus, although wanting assistance, persons may find it difficult to relinquish responsibilities. This jeopardizes their own well-being as well as relationships with others seeking more involvement. Among siblings, stress can occur when one resents another's lack of involvement or when one minimizes the other's contributions (Ingersoll-Dayton, Neal, Ha, & Hammer, 2003).

Employment and Caregiving

Balancing employment with caregiving can be particularly challenging, and especially taxing for women who continue to be the primary caregivers. The typical caregiver is a 46-year-old employed married woman earning an annual income of $35,000 (National Alliance of Caregiving and American Association of Retired Persons, 1997). These women are often providing care for their own children while struggling to meet the dual demands of work and care for a parent. The impact on women employees is noted in one study that found employed women caregivers reporting more depression than employed men caregivers (Lee, Walker, & Shoup, 2001). Compounding these demands is financial strain, as one study found that 49% of these midlife women suffered financial hardship as a result of their caregiving (National Alliance of Caregiving and American Association of Retired Persons, 1997). The effects of caregiving on women's employment and financial well-being were highlighted in a national study of elder care (Metropolitan Life Insurance Company, 1999):

- 33% of working women decreased their work hours
- 29% passed up a job promotion, training, or assignment
- 22% took a leave of absence to provide care
- 20% switched from full-time to part-time employment
- 16% left their employment
- 13% took early retirement

It is evident that caregiving can have a serious impact on both a woman's present and future financial status, since it affects not only present income but also contributions to both private pensions and Social Security. In addition, research has found that once caregiving stops, women do not increase their employment, suggesting that the work time lost during caregiving is not easily recovered (Pavalko & Artis, 1997). Those who do return to work after caregiving are likely to receive lower wages, have fewer employment–related benefits, and receive reduced retirement benefits (Dettinger & Clarkberg, 2002).

Caregiving ramifications extend to the employer as well. A study made by Transamerica Life Insurance Company found that one and a half times as many caregivers than non-caregivers reported missing work or having to take time off due to family responsibilities. Other research reports the cost for businesses to replace women who left in order to provide care is estimated at $3.3 billion per year, while absenteeism due to caregiving responsibilities has been estimated at $270 million (Metropolitan Life and National Association of Caregiving, 1997).

CAREGIVER STATUS

Much has been written about the impact of caregiving responsibilities on the physical and mental health status of the caregiver and the burden and stress they may encounter. One model for understanding the effects of caregiving is based on the caregiver's cognitive appraisal of the situation, as this influences both the stress and coping of the caregiver (Gatz, Bengston, & Blum, 1990).

Caregiver stress can also be caused by a series of primary and secondary stressors. Primary stressors are the difficulties associated with caregiving and secondary the role strains and changes in self-concepts (Pearlin, Mullan, Semple, & Skaff, 1990). The caregiver's perception of role overload is fundamental in this process, with overload defined as feeling exhausted, not having enough time for oneself and the caregiving tasks, and the feeling that there is no progress in the caregiving relationship. Role overload is viewed as particularly harmful to caregiver well-being (Skaff & Pearlin, 1992).

Caregiver to an older adult has become a common adult role, but it remains one for which there is little preparation and one that can place incomparable demands for time and energy. For many, it severely alters their own lives as it competes with their existing roles and future plans. On the other hand, for some, caregiving has very positive effects in their lives. Feeling useful and involved in a positive role, feeling appreciated, and having the opportunity to express feelings of love and intimacy to the care recipient are among positive aspects (Bass, 1990; Aneshensel, Pearlin, Mullan, Zarit, & Whitlatch, 1995). Moreover, when it becomes a meaningful relationship, caregivers are likely to feel greater self-esteem and to be less depressed (Noonan & Tennstedt, 1997).

Though caregiving can have positive effects, research continues to underscore its negative effects on many measures of well-being. In a review of research detailing differences between caregivers and non-caregivers, caregivers were continually found to be more impaired in measures of psychological and physical health, with the largest differences found in depression, stress, self-efficacy, and subjective well-being (Pinquart & Sorenson, 2003). In addition, the greatest differences were noted between dementia caregivers and non-caregivers.

Many factors appear to be associated with individuals' responses to caregiving. Personality is one characteristic that may influence the ability to adapt to the role. It may in fact be more important than losses in predicting stress and a spousal caregiver's physical and mental health (Hooker, Monahan, Bowman, Frazier, & Shifrin, 1998). Other research on spousal caregivers shows their health generally deteriorating, and those moving into heavier caregiving tasks report more depression, poorer health, and poorer health behaviors (Burton et al., 2003).

Research on gender differences and caregiving find women more likely than men to report negative effects when caring for either a spouse or a parent (Cannuscio, Jones, Kawachi, Colditz, Berkman, & Rimm, 2002). In comparison with non-caregiving wives, those caring for a disabled spouse were six times as likely to report anxiety or depressive symptoms. In addition, older women are twice as likely as older men to receive assistance (Davey et al., 1999). At the same time, women are among those most likely to report that their care is inadequate, suggesting that they may place greater demands on caregivers (Lima & Allen, 2001). Divorced or separated persons have the smallest network of helpers and are thus at risk of not having their needs met (Barrett & Lynch, 1999).

Other findings (Given, Given, Stommel, & Assouz, 1999) underscore the complexity of the caregiving relationship, as male caregivers are more likely to report higher levels of depressive symptoms over time, with this depression unrelated to deterioration in the relative's status. These findings suggest that the amount, type, and duration of caregiver assistance may be more important than gender in predicting well-being. In addition, caregivers living with the relative experience higher levels of burden than those maintaining separate households (Hughes, Giobbi-Hurder, Weaver, Kubal, & Henderson, 1999; Knight, Williams, McGee, & Olaman, 1998), while those not living with the relative report feeling more worried (Cox & Albisu, 2003).

Caring for persons with dementia is particularly stressful due to demands resulting from the care receiver's problematic and erratic behavior. Although the cognitively impaired may not require direct physical interventions, they typically need constant supervision and direction, and this can be even more time-consuming and mentally exhausting than physical assistance. At the same time, the prognosis is usually poor, that is, both continued mental and physical deterioration are expected, causing further worry and stress to the caregiver. Additionally, persons with dementia are frequently nonresponsive to assistance or actually resist it, in some instances accusing the caregiver of intentional harm. With the progression of the illness, caregiver strength and feelings of mastery can be severely challenged (Bauer, Maddox, Kirk, Burns, & Kuskowski, 2001).

Data from a national survey comparing caregivers of persons with Alzheimer's disease with other caregivers finds the former providing more hours of care per week and providing more intense and involved care (Alzheimer's Association and Alliance for Caregiving, 1999). They are also less likely to feel that other relatives are providing sufficient assistance and to report some family conflict over this involvement. With regard to their own status, they are twice as likely as other caregivers to report a physical or mental health problem as a result of their caregiving.

INFORMAL AND FORMAL NETWORKS

There has been ongoing policy concern that the introduction of formal services in the care of an impaired older person will displace informal assistance by the family. The concern appears rooted in traditional ideologies that emphasize the importance of independence and autonomy as well as family responsibility and obligations. However, existing data gives little credibility to concerns that family values and involvement will be eroded by the introduction of formal services into the caregiving system.

Litwak (1985) stresses the complementary nature of formal-informal relationships. The informal is best suited for unpredictable, nontechnical tasks associated with care, while the formal system can better deal with specialized tasks. According to this model, these two systems are not substitutable. The informal system is best able to provide the emotional support or assistance during a crisis. The formal system may be best able to cope with the highly skilled or arduous aspects of caregiving.

Noelker and Bass (1989) present evidence that formal services may play both a supplementary and complementary role depending on the characteristics of the caregiver. Formal services to supplement assistance are likely to be used by female caregivers. Males and those caring for the very impaired are more likely to use formal services for specialized care. Furthermore, caregiver needs, rather than those of the relative, appear to be the main determinants of service use for all caregivers. Thus, caregivers who are themselves frail or have had changes in their health are more likely to use formal services regardless of the condition of the frail relative.

Caregivers apparently do not turn to formal services until they are no longer able to meet caregiving demands. It is thus not surprising that both their physical and mental health may suffer and actually deteriorate as a result of the caregiving tasks. Rather than using interventions as preventive and support measures, they are used as remedial ones when the primary caregiver finds coping difficult (Cox & Monk, 1990). Even in these instances, such services do not appear to substitute for informal care.

Studies reporting reductions in informal care with the use of formal services have found that reductions were slight. Moreover, the reductions did not impact on the assistance provided by family but involved only that provided by friends and neighbors, and even this reduction was temporary (Christianson, 1988). Other research shows no permanent reduction in informal care with the introduction of formal services (Tennstedt, Crawford, & McKinlay, 1993; Tennstedt, Harrow, & Crawford, 1996).

In an examination of both informal care and self-care by older persons with chronic illness, not only was it found that the greater use of formal services did not cause a reduction in informal care, but it also did not reduce the older person's efforts for self-care (Penning, 2002). The number of chronic conditions and levels of functional and cognitive impairment were most closely related to both types of care, with the extent of formal care received showing no substitution for either type of care.

CAREGIVER SUPPORTS

The National Family Caregiver Support Program was instituted as part of the Older Americans Act in 2000 and is administered by the Administration on Aging. The goal of the act is to help states develop services and service networks that can meet the needs of older persons and the caregivers on whom they depend. Grants are given to states on a formula based on their 70-and-older population.

In the allocation of funds, priority is to be given to those with the greatest social and economic needs, with particular attention given to low-income, minority persons, and older persons caring for those with mental retardation and related developmental disabilities. The funds are allocated to five direct services: caregiver information; assistance accessing supportive services; individual counseling; organization of support groups, and caregiver training, respite care, and supplemental services that complement caregiver support.

The National Family Caregiver Support Program is critically important as a first step in national recognition of the role that the family plays in supporting seniors and their needs for assistance. It is noteworthy in the emphasis it gives to the family as a dyad, and the ways in which relatives are intimately involved in the care of relatives as well as their needs for assistance. In addition to providing some support to the family, it affirms the desire of older persons to remain in the community as long as possible.

However, with its careful targeting on those in the greatest social and economic need, and with the average caregiver earning $35,000 annually (National Alliance of Caregiving and American Association of

Retired Persons, 1997), millions of family caregivers in need of assistance remain outside of the program's parameters. In addition, restricted funding of the legislation limits the extent to which the act can sufficiently meet the needs of those who are eligible for services.

INTERVENTIONS

In designing interventions to assist caregivers, it is important to recognize that varying factors can affect both use and effectiveness. A summary of findings on interventions from several studies found that offering psychoeducational interventions and psychotherapy were effective in improving caregiver well-being and increasing knowledge and ability in the short term (Sorensen, Pinquart, Habil, & Duberstein, 2002). The results also indicated that group interventions may be less effective than individual ones in reducing caregiver depression and increasing well-being, but that groups were more effective in improving care receiver symptoms. Age was important in offering interventions, with older caregivers more likely to benefit from services offering them more relief from caregiving or giving emotional support. Women showed more benefit from interventions than men; adult children benefited more than spouses.

Two specific services focusing on needs of family caregivers are support groups and respite care. Both types focus on offering assistance to caregivers to relieve and strengthen them in their caregiving roles, and both have become widely available in varying forms throughout the country.

Support Groups

Support groups function to assist caregivers in coping with stresses associated with their roles through the sharing of mutual emotional support and information. These groups provide settings in which caregivers can discuss their concerns and problems with others in the same situations. Simultaneously, members can learn from each other new ways of dealing with specific problems. The groups are also important means for counteracting the isolation that caregivers frequently experience. In fact, many groups encourage members to exchange telephone numbers and to meet outside of the group, often sharing caregiving tasks and relieving each other.

Many support groups focus on specific medical problems or illnesses such as strokes, heart attacks, or dementia. This type of group enables the caregivers to better identify with the problems faced by the group members and thus to offer mutual empathy and assistance. Being able to ventilate frustrations with those dealing with similar illnesses can assist in creating a sense of solidarity that is fundamental to meeting support needs.

The significant role support groups can play is indicated by the fact that participation in such groups can deter the use of nursing homes. Greene and Monahan (1987) found that frail relatives of family caregivers participating in support and education groups had significantly lower rates of placement in nursing homes than the frail relatives of comparable caregivers not participating in such groups. The groups permitted participants to deal with negative feelings, overcome the sense of emotional isolation, and share difficult experiences as well as effective problem-solving techniques. Each meeting involved education on particular skills such as moving, bathing, and lifting. Finally, the sessions also included relaxation training and stress-reduction techniques.

In a thorough review of family support groups, however, Toseland, Rossiter, and Lebreque (1989) find that group outcomes may actually be more limited. Many studies have not really measured the effectiveness of such groups in reducing caregivers' sense of burden and level of stress. Although most participants evaluate the group experience positively, reporting such gains as new insight and the development of a sense of community, it is difficult to establish a link between such programs and the development of new coping skills or the alleviation of psychological problems.

A key limitation to the effectiveness of such groups is the tendency for family members to not attend them until stress is already quite severe. Reaching families in earlier stages of an illness may be an important part in the coping process. However, the very families who may best benefit from such programs may also have the most difficulties committing to the programs. Caregiving responsibilities that contribute to the need for support may also act as barriers to participation (Cox, 1997).

Respite Care

Respite care offers relief from caregiving either through in-home respite, adult day care, or overnight respite. By offering caregivers temporary relief, respite attempts to improve caregiver well-being, primarily by decreasing feelings of burden and stress.

In-home respite is the most preferred type of care and widely used. Among the benefits associated with respite are improved mood, less emotional stress, and less burden (Cox, 1997; Curran, 1995). Caregiver satisfaction with the programs has been associated with their expectations, service access, and the ease of obtaining the service (Townsend & Koslowski, 2002).

Although caregivers may seek the service, however, it is often difficult to get them to commit to the program (Cox, 1997; Montgomery, 1988). In addition, many stop using the service after only a few months, placing their relative in a nursing home, possibly due to the fact that they turn to respite when the relative is already quite impaired and the small amount of help they receive is not sufficient to relieve them. Users of in-home respite may be concerned over the training of the workers, their reliability, and the agency itself (Malone-Beach, Zarit, & Spore, 1992; Montgomery, 1995).

In order to assure the most effective use of respite it is important to reach caregivers earlier in the caregiving process. Equally important is providing persons with a sufficient amount of care so that the amount of time that they spend in caregiving tasks is actually reduced. Identifying the type of respite, whether in-home or out of home, that would best meet the needs of the caregiver may also help to improve both utilization and program outcomes. No less important is assuring that the respite providers are competent in caring for older persons as well as in dealing with caregiver concerns.

SUMMARY

Families are the main providers of community care for older persons, with women, primarily adult daughters, comprising the majority. Caregiving tends to follow a continuum with persons turning first to their spouses and then to adult children and other relatives. Many factors influence the caregiving relationship, including feelings of reciprocity, commitment, affection, values, and norms. Even distant relatives may assume the caregiving role.

Many theories and models have been developed that explain caregiving and the caregiving relationship. Most models have focused on its negative effects on caregivers and the factors contributing to caregiver stress and well-being. At the same time, it is important to recognize the positive aspects of caregiving. It can increase self-esteem, feelings of being appreciated, and the ability of the caregiver to express feelings of love and intimacy.

Most attention has focused on the stress of caregivers in their attempts to meet the needs of their relative as well as other demands. In particular, stress is most likely to occur in those caring for persons with dementia whose needs for care continue increasing regardless of the caregiver's involvement. As these demands escalate, caregivers are at risk of experiencing both physical and mental problems.

Stress is likely to occur as persons find themselves struggling to meet the needs of their relative as well as other demands. Employed caregivers face particular burdens as they try to balance caregiving responsibilities with those of work. The impact is felt by both employees and employers, through high rates of absenteeism, lower wages, and reduced benefits.

Caregivers of relatives with dementia are particularly vulnerable as needs for care continue to escalate with the disease. The problematic and erratic behavior of the relative and need for constant supervision can severely tax caregiver coping abilities. The relative's resistance to care or inability to express appreciation can cause further stress.

Caregivers continue to use only limited formal services to assist them. Interventions tend to be used as remedial rather than preventive measures. Most turn to the formal sector only when the demands for care become severe and they are experiencing difficulty coping. At the same time, there is no evidence that the use of formal services actually decreases family involvement or the individual's efforts at self-care.

The National Family Caregivers Support Program marks the first real attempt by the federal government to provide support to caregivers. The program recognizes the roles these persons play, but with its targeting of those with the greatest need and its limited funding, its ability to truly provide support remains in doubt. Other important interventions are support groups, which can assist persons in dealing with the stress of caregiving as well as teach them new skills; and respite care that can offer real relief from the caregiving role. However, the effectiveness of each of these interventions depends to a large measure upon their design, and their abilities to reach those caregivers that might derive the greatest benefits from them.

REFERENCES

Agency for Healthcare Research and Quality. (2001). *The characteristics of long-term care users.* AHRQ Research Report, AHRQ Publication No. 00-0049. Rockville, MD: Author.

Alzheimer's Association and Alliance for Caregiving. (1999). *Who cares? Families caring for persons with Alzheimer's disease.* Washington, DC: Alzheimer's Association.

Aneshensel, C., Pearlin, L., Mullan, J., Zarit, S., & Whitlach, C. (1995). *Profiles in caregiving: The unexpected career.* San Diego: Academic Press.

Antonnucci, T., & Depner, C. (1982). Social support and informal helping relationships. In T. A. Wills (Ed.), *Basic processes in helping relationships.* New York: Academic Press.

Barrett, A., & Lynch, S. (1999). Caregiving networks of elderly persons: Variations by marital status. *Gerontologist, 39,* 695–704.

Bass, D. (1990). *Caring families: Supports and interventions.* Silver Spring, MD: NASW Press.

Bauer, M., Maddox, M., Kirk, L., Burns, T., & Kuskowski, M. (2001). Progressive dementia: Personal and relational impact on caregiving wives. *American Journal of Alzheimer's Disease and Other Dementia, 16,* 329–334.

Beisgen, B., & Kritchman, M. (2003). *Senior centers: Opportunities for successful aging.* New York: Springer Publishing.

Bengston, V., Rosenthal, C., & Burton, L. (1996). Paradoxes of families and aging. In R. Binstock & L. George (Eds.), *Handbook of aging and the social sciences* (4th ed.). New York: Academic Press.

Brody, E., Hoffman, C., Kleban, M., & Schoonhover, C. (1989). Caregiving daughters and their local siblings: Perceptions, strains, and interactions. *Gerontologist, 29,* 529–538.

Burton, L., Zdaniuk, B., Schulz, R., Jackson, R., & Hirsch, C. (2003). Transitions in spousal caregiving. *Gerontologist, 43,* 230–241.

Cannuscio, C., Jones, C., Kawachi, I., Colditz, G., Berkman, L., & Rimm, E. (2002). Reverberations of family illness: A longitudinal assessment of informal caregiving and mental health status in the Nurses' Health Study. *American Journal of Public Health, 92,* 1305–1311.

Chodorow, N. (1978). *The reproduction of mothering: Psychoanalysis and the sociology of gender.* Berkeley: University of California Press.

Christianson, J. (1988). The evaluation of the national long-term care demonstration: 6. The effect of channeling on informal caregiving. *Health Services Research, 23*(1), entire issue.

Connadis, I., Rosenthal, C., & McMullin, J. (1996). The impact of family composition on providing help to older parents: A study of employed adults. *Research on Aging, 18,* 402–429.

Coward, R., Horne, C., & Dwyer, J. (1992). Demographic perspectives on gender and family. In J. W. Dwyer & R. T. Coward (Eds.), *Gender, families, and elder care* (pp. 18–33). Newbury Park, CA: Sage.

Cox, C. (1997). Findings from a statewide program of respite care: A comparison of service users, stoppers, and non-users. *Gerontologist, 37,* 511–517.

Cox, C., & Albisu, K. (2003). The impact of caring for a relative with dementia: A comparison of those caring for persons living alone, spousal caregivers, and co-resident adult children. *Journal of Mental Health and Aging, 8,* 216–230.

Cox, C., & Monk, A. (1990). Minority caregivers of dementia victims: A comparison of Black and Hispanic families. *Journal of Applied Gerontology, 9,* 340–354.

Curran, J. (1995). Current provision and effectiveness of day care services for people with dementia. *Reviews in Clinical Gerontology, 5,* 313–320.

Davey, A., Femia, E., Shea, D., Zarit, S., Sundstrom, G., Berg, S., & Smyer, M. (1999). How many elders receive assistance? *Journal of Aging and Health, 11,* 199–220.

Dettinger, E., & Clarksberg, M. (2002). Informal caregiving and retirement timing among men and women: Gender and caregiving. *Journal of Family Issues, 23*(7), 857–879.

Dowd, J. (1980). *Stratification among the aged.* Monterey, CA: Brooks/Cole.

Freedman, V. (1996). Family structure and the risk of nursing home admission. *Journal of Gerontology: Social Sciences, 51B*(2), S61–S69

Gallant, M., & Connell, C. (1997). Predictors of decreased self-care among spouse caregivers of older adults with dementing illnesses. *Journal of Aging and Health, 9,* 373–395.

Gatz, M., Bengston, V., & Blum, M. (1990). Caregiving families. In J. Birren & K. Schaie (Eds.), *Handbook of the psychology of aging* (3rd ed.). San Diego: Academic Press.

Given, C., Given, B., Stommel, M., & Assouz, F. (1999). The impact of new demands for assistance on caregiver depression: Tests using an inception cohort. *Gerontologist, 39,* 76–85.

Greene, V., & Monahan, D. (1987). The effect of a professionally guided caregiver support and education group on institutionalization of care receivers. *Gerontologist, 27,* 716–722.

Hooker, K., Monahan, D., Bowman, S., Frazier, L., & Shifrin, K. (1998). Personality counts for a lot: Predictors of mental and physical health of spouse caregivers in two disease groups. *Journal of Gerontology, Psychological Sciences, 53B,* P73–P85.

Horowitz, A. (1985). Family caregiving to the frail elderly. In C. Eisdorfer (Ed.), *Annual review of gerontology and geriatrics* (pp. 194–246). New York: Springer Publishing.

Hooyman, N. (1999). Research on older women; Where is feminism? *Gerontologist, 39,* 115–118.

Hughes, S., Giobbie-Hurder, A., Weaver, F., Kubal, J., & Henderson, W. (1999). Relationship between caregiver burden and health-related quality of life. *Gerontologist, 39,* 534–545.

Ingersoll-Dayton, B., Neal, M., Ha, J., & Hammer, L. (2003). Redressing inequity in parent care among siblings. *Journal of Marriage and the Family, 65,* 201–212.

Katz, S. (2000). Disabled elderly women receive less home care than men. *Journal of the American Medical Association, 284,* 3022–3027.

Knight, R., Williams, S., McGee, R., & Olaman, S. (1998). Caregiving and well-being in a sample of women in midlife. *Australian and New Zealand Journal of Public Health, 22,* 616–620.

Kramer, B. (1997). Differential predictors of strain and gain among husbands caring for wives with dementia. *Gerontologist, 37,* 239–249.

Laditka, J., & Laditka, S. (2000). Aging children and their older parents: The coming generation of caregiving *Journal of Women and Aging, 12,* 189–204.

Lee, P. (1985). Theoretical perspectives on social networks. In W. Sauer & R. Coward (Eds.), *Social support networks and the care of the elderly.* New York: Springer Publishing.

Lee, G., Dwyer, J., & Coward, R. (1993). Gender differences in parent care: Demographic factors and same-gender preferences. *Journal of Gerontology, Social Sciences, 48,* S9–S16.

Lee, G., & Ellithorpe, E. (1982). Intergenerational and subjective well being among the elderly. *Journal of Marriage and the Family, 44,* 217–224.

Lee, J., Walker, M., & Shoup, R. (2001). Balancing elder care responsibilities and work: The impact on emotional health. *Journal of Business and Psychology, 16,* 277–289.

Liang, J., Krause, N., & Bennett, J. (2001). Social exchange and well-being: Is giving better than receiving? *Psychology and Aging, 16,* 511–523.

Lima, J., & Allen, S. (2001). Targeting risk for unmet need: Not enough help versus no help at all. *Journal of Gerontology, Social Sciences, 56B,* S302–S310.

Litwak, E. (1985). *Helping the elderly: The complementary roles of informal networks and formal systems.* New York: Guilford.

Lyons, K., Zarit, S., Sayer, C., & Whitlatch, C. (2002). Caregiving as a dyadic process. *Journal of Gerontology, Psychological Sciences and Social Sciences, 57,* P195–P204.

Marks, N., Lambert, J., & Choi, H. (2002). Transitions to caregiving: Gender and psychological well-being—a prospective U.S. national survey. *Journal of Marriage and the Family, 64,* 657–667.

Metropolitan Life Insurance Company & National Alliance for Caregivers. (1997). *The Metlife study of employer costs for working caregivers.* Westport, CT: Metropolitan Life Insurance Company.

Metropolitan Life Insurance Company, Study of Employer Costs for Working Caregivers. (1999). *The Metlife juggling act study: Balancing caregiving with work and the costs involved.* Westport, CT: Metlife.

Malone-Beach, E., Zarit, S., & Spore, D. (1992). Caregivers' perceptions of case management and community-based services: Barriers to service use. *Journal of Applied Gerontology, 11,* 146–159.

Montgomery, R. (1988). Respite care: Lessons from a controlled design study. *Health Care Financing Review,* Annual Supplement, 133–138.

Montgomery, R. (1995). Examining respite care: Promises and limitations. In R. Kane & J. Perod (Eds.), *Family caregiving in an aging society* (pp. 22–45). London: Sage.

Mutran, E., & Reitzes, D. (1984). Intergenerational support activities and well-being among the elderly: A convergence of exchange and symbolic interaction perspectives. *American Sociological Review, 49,* 117–130.

Naivaie-Waliser, M., Spriggs, A., & Feldman, P. (2002). Informal caregiving: Differential experiences by gender. *Medical Care, 40,* 1249–1259.

National Alliance of Caregiving and American Association of Retired Persons. (1997). *Family caregiving in the United States: Findings from a national study.* Washington, DC: American Association of Retired Persons.

Noelker, L., & Bass, D. (1989). Home care for elderly persons: Linkages between formal and informal caregivers. *Journal of Gerontology, 44,* 563–570.

Noonan, A., & Tennstedt, S. (1997). Meaning in caregiving and its contribution to caregiver well-being. *Gerontologist, 37,* 785–794.

Pavalko, E., & Artis, J. (1997). Women's caregiving and paid work: Causal relationships in late life. *Journal of Gerontology: Social Sciences, 52B*(4), 170–179.

Pearlin, L., Mullan, J., Semple, S., & Skaff, M. (1990). Caregiving and the stress process: An overview of concepts and their measures. *Gerontologist, 30,* 583–591.

Penning, M. (2002). Hydra revisited: Substituting formal for self- and informal in-home care among older adults with disabilities. *Gerontologist, 42,* 4–16.

Penrod, J., Kane, R., Kane, R., & Finch, M. (1995). Who cares? The size, scope, and composition of the caregiver support system. *Gerontologist, 35,* 485–497.

Pinquart, M., & Sorenson, S. (2003). Differences between caregivers and non-caregivers in psychological health and physical health: A meta-analysis. *Psychology and Aging, 18,* 250–267.

Pruchno, R., Burant, C., & Peters, N. (1997). Typologies of caregiving families: Congruence and individual well-being. *Gerontologist, 37,* 157–167.

Ray, R. (1999). A postmodern perspective on feminist gerontology. *Gerontologist 36,* 674–680.

Roberts, R., & Bengston, V. (1990). Is intergenerational solidarity a unidimensional construct? A second test of a formal model. *Journal of Gerontology, 45,* S12–S20.

Schone, B., & Pezzin, L. (1999). Divorce reduces informal caregiving and economic ties between elderly parents and their adult children. *Demography, 36,* 287–297.

Seltzer, M., & Wailing Li, L. (1996). The transitions of caregiving: Subjective and objective definitions. *Gerontologist, 36,* 614–626.

Shulz, R., & Beach, S. (1999). Caregiving as a risk factor for mortality: The Caregiver Health Effects Study. *Journal of the American Medical Association, 282,* 2215–2219.

Skaff, M., & Pearlin, L. (1992). Caregiving: Role engulfment and the loss of self. *Gerontologist, 32,* 656–664.

Soldo, B., Agree, E., & Wolf, D. (1989). The balance between formal and informal care. In M. Ory & K. Bond (Eds.), *Aging and health care: Social science and policy perspectives* (pp. 193–216). London: Routledge.

Sorensen, S., Pinquart, M., Habil, D., & Duberstein, P. (2002). How effective are interventions with caregivers? An updated meta-analysis. *Gerontologist, 42,* 356–372.

Spillman, P., & Pezzin, L. (2000). Potential and active family caregivers: Changing networks and the sandwich generation. *Milbank Quarterly, 78,* 347–374.

Spitze, G., & Logan, J. (1990). Sons, daughters, and intergenerational support. *Journal of Marriage and the Family, 52,* 420–430.

Stephens, S., & Christianson, J. (1986). *Informal care of the elderly.* Lexington, MA: Lexington Books.

Stoller, E. (1985). Exchange patterns in the informal networks of the elderly: The impact of reciprocity on morale. *Journal of Marriage and the Family, 47,* 335–342.

Stoller, E. (1994). Gender and the organization of lay health care: A socialist-feminist perspective. *Journal of Aging Studies, 7,* 151–170.

Stoller, E., & Pugliesi, K. (1991). Informal networks of community-based elderly. *Research on Aging, 10,* 499–516.

Stone, R. (2000). *Long term care for the elderly with disabilities: Current policy, emerging trends, and implications for the twenty-first century.* New York: Milbank Memorial Fund.

Talbott, M. (1990). The negative side of the relationship between older widows and their adult children: The mothers' perspective. *Gerontologist, 30,* 595–603.

Tennstedt, S., Crawford, S., & McKinlay, J. (1993). Is family care on the decline: A longitudinal investigation of the substitution of formal long-term care services for informal care. *Milbank Quarterly, 71,* 601–624.

Tennstedt, S., Harrow, B., & Crawford, S. (1996). Informal care versus formal services: Changes in patterns of care over time. *Journal of Aging and Social Policy, 7,* 71–91.

Toseland, R. W., Rossiter, C. M., & Lebreque, M. S. (1989). The effectiveness of peer led and professionally led groups to support family caregivers. *Gerontologist, 29*(4), 465–471.

Townsend, D., & Koslowski, K. (2002). Factors related to client satisfaction with community-based respite services. *Home Health Services Quarterly, 21,* 89–106.

Willliamson, G., & Shaffer, R. (2001). Relationship quality and potentially harmful behaviors by spousal caregivers: How we were then and how we are now. *Psychology and Aging, 16,* 217–226.

Wolf, D., Freedman, V., & Soldo, B. (1997). The division of family labor: Care for elderly parents. *Journal of Gerontology, Social Sciences, 52B,* 102–109.

Young, R., & Kahana, E. (1989). Specifying caregiver outcomes: Gender and relationship aspects of caregiving strain. *Gerontologist, 29,* 660–666.

Chapter 7

Ethnicity and Care

Deciding when care is needed, who should provide it, and how it should be offered is a multifaceted decision. The response is determined not only by the older person's impairment or disability level, but also by the values, traditions, and culture of the group to which the senior belongs. Among the critical factors that can influence the perception and development of frailty is ethnicity. In fact, ethnicity, because it relates to the individual's role in society and interactions with others, provides the context in which factors such as gender, family, and the use of services are organized.

It is critical to remember that culture itself is not a constant and that adherence to ethnic values and traditions varies with many other factors. Ethnicity remains a very complex phenomenon that can be affected by birthplace, years after immigration and assimilation. Viewing each particular group, subgroup, and even family in terms of its own unique background and experiences is essential in understanding responses to impairments and to needs for care.

Ethnicity encompasses a distinct way of viewing and reacting to the world. Race, religion, or national origin are markers of ethnicity, with individual members classified according to the degree to which they identify with a specific group as well as the extent to which others consider them to be "ethnic" (Shibutani & Kwan, 1965).

Ethnic groups commonly hold distinct cultural beliefs, values, and norms. These can influence the aging process, determining the ways in which individuals are expected to age, their status, and their relationships, including the ways in which persons should care for and be involved with the those who become impaired. As important as ethnicity may be as a critical influence on the care of older persons, it is not a constant force. Age, acculturation, and socioeconomic status contribute to the saliency of ethnicity as a force in a person's life (Markides, Liang, & Jackson, 1990).

Given the fact that ethnic culture and attitudes can affect care, it is imperative to recognize that ethnic disparities also exist within the caregiving network. Studies continue to show that professionals and systems maintain biases and discriminatory attitudes that affect services received by minority elders (White-Means, 2000; Johnson & Smith, 2002). According to the Institute of Medicine (2002), racial and ethnic minorities in the United States receive lower quality care than non-minority Whites. Among the factors contributing to this disparity are clinical uncertainty, stereotypical behavior, and conscious bias that can extend to prejudice.

IMPAIRMENT AND ETHNICITY

The prevalence of chronic diseases varies by race and ethnicity. Black and Hispanic elderly have higher levels of diabetes than White non-Hispanics, with Black elderly also having much higher rates of hypertension (National Center for Health Statistics, 1999). The same data also show Black elderly as reporting more limitations in their activities and being more likely to have difficulties performing activities of daily living than White elderly. Other national data (Carrasquillo, Lantigua, & Shea, 2000) show Hispanic elders as having similar levels of ADL and IADL dependencies as White non-Hispanics, with Blacks again having the highest level of impairments and requiring the use of assistive devices.

Data on differences in cognitive impairment indicate greater rates of impairment among Hispanic elders than among other groups (Gurland et al., 1997; Tang et al., 1998; Carasquillo et al., 2000). Studies also indicate that compared with White non-Hispanic elderly, Hispanics have lower rates of Alzheimer's disease but higher rates of vascular dementia (Fritz, Ortiz, & Ponton, 2001). Puerto Ricans have been found to be more disabled than Blacks or Whites with the disability beginning early in life and continuing into old age. In addition, variations among subgroups of ethnic populations are also apparent. In comparison with Mexican Americans and Cuban Americans, Puerto Rican elderly have greater levels of disability (Burnette & Mui, 1995).

RESPONSES TO IMPAIRMENT

As ethnicity influences one's view of the world, it may also influence the perception of impairment. Disabilities or impairments that limit an older person's functioning may be perceived as an expected part of the normal course of aging. Within this perspective, an impairment may be accepted as a natural occurrence and not perceived as a symbol of decline or dependency. Older persons will not perceive themselves as dependent if they are able to provide some type of support or assistance to other family members.

This type of exchange or mutual assistance, whether financial, emotional, hands-on, or even symbolic, promotes the older person's sense of self-esteem and connectedness while permitting him or her to continue to play a role within the family (Becker, Beyee, Newsom, & Mayem, 2003). The importance of social roles in responses to impairment is further underscored by research showing that maintaining roles and some personal control assists older person adapt to declines in health, and actually reduces disability (Seeman, Baker, Richardson, & Tinetti, 1996). For example, if older persons are depended upon for child care or other assistance, they are less likely to identify themselves as disabled or impaired.

However, though these attitudes and behaviors may assist in adaptation, they may also affect the decision to seek care. In some instances, as the person feels responsible for some aspect of the family's well-being, he or she may deny his/her own need for care. The result is that care is sought only when the illness or impairment has become significantly disabling. In addition, older persons who feel responsible for assisting the family may deny their own impairments in order to continue in their traditional roles.

Responses of ethnic groups to cognitive impairments in the elderly warrant specific attention. Frequently, dementia is not recognized by families that regard cognitive deficits and behavioral problems as a normal part of aging. Ethnic groups assign meaning to dementia according to their own values, norms, and beliefs, which further influence their own caregiving activities as well as their use of services. Thus, to the extent that families are accepting of cognitive impairments in their older relatives, they are less likely to seek medical care and treatment for symptoms. Therefore, many remain at risk of not receiving medications that can slow the course of illness or help reduce symptoms.

At the same time, it is critical that any attempt to understand a group's responses to impairments considers the social milieu and environment in which the persons live. Thus, histories of poor access to care, inadequate services, and culturally insensitive providers can affect the older person's responses to symptoms and impairments, particularly his or her proclivity to seek formal assistance. In addition, little knowledge or education regarding the nature of impairments or appropriate treatments can further affect the ways persons respond.

AFRICAN AMERICANS

As discussed earlier, African American elderly, compared with other groups, are more likely to have functional impairments and difficulties with the activities of daily living. The population rates their health as more poor than either White or Hispanic elderly (Benson & Marano, 1998). As well as being more likely to have life-threatening illnesses such as heart disease and hypertension, they also have high rates of arthritis, which can severely restrict mobility. In addition, African American elderly are more likely to report being ill and to be disabled at an earlier age than their White peers.

At the same time, older Black persons are less likely to receive appropriate health care services than White elderly. Often they lack access to such care as screenings, physical and occupational therapies that may be available to other groups due to a lack of knowledge about techniques, limited income, and limited insurance. Given the low income status of many Black elderly, a reliance on Medicaid and Medicare, and their concentrations in urban centers, they often lack access to physicians who can assist them in receiving such services and thus race becomes a key factor in explaining the use of community health care (White-Means, 2000). In addition, when they do receive medical care, they receive lower-cost procedures and services, even under Medicare (Lee, Gehlbach, Hosmer, Reti, & Baker, 1997).

Studies on the use of home care services by older African Americans have found varying results. Whereas some studies indicate the group uses less home care than older non-Hispanic Whites (Mui & Burnette, 1994; Wallace, Levy-Storms, Kingston, & Andersen, 1998), others find that race does not affect use and that any differences that do occur are dependent on income and Medicaid status (Miller et al., 1996).

HISPANICS

Data from the 1999 Medical Expenditures Panel Survey is used to describe the health of Hispanics aged 50 years and older (Center for an Aging Society, 2003). The data reveal that the proportion of older Hispanics having at least one chronic condition is similar to that of non-Hispanic Whites. However, Hispanics are less likely than other groups to see a physician or to use other health care providers such as optometrists, psychologists, chiropractors, physical therapists, occupational therapists, or social workers.

Less than one third of older Hispanics with chronic conditions had insurance coverage for prescription drugs, compared with 39% of non-Hispanic Blacks and 52% of non-Hispanic Whites. Hispanics are also more likely to be either uninsured (27%) or dependent on Medicaid (24%) than the other groups. For those over the age of 65, more than one third are dependent solely on public programs (i.e., Medicaid and Medicare) for their health care. Only 20% of Hispanics, compared to 31% of non-Hispanic Blacks and 60% of non-Hispanic Whites, have Medicare and private insurance.

The disparities in health care for Hispanics with chronic disease are also noted in their use of preventive and maintenance services. In comparison to other groups with diabetes, hypertension, or heart disease, older Hispanics are less likely than either non-Hispanic Whites or Blacks to have their conditions regularly monitored. The group also reports more difficulty in making appointments with their health care providers and not surprisingly, tends to be less satisfied with their care.

Disparities in health care seriously affect the functioning of older Hispanics. For instance, data indicate that this group is much less likely to have hip replacements, even under Medicare, than non-Hispanic Whites suffering from the same arthritic condition (Escalante et al., 2002). Accordingly, these persons continue to be in pain and their impaired functioning leads to greater dependency. The lack of surgery reflects a lack of familiarity with the procedure and difficulties in communicating with the physician.

ASIAN PACIFIC ISLANDERS

Asian Pacific Islander elderly are the second-fastest growing older population in the United States. Projections of future growth indicate that by 2050 Asian Americans will compose 6.3% of the older population, in comparison with 9.3% Blacks and 17.5% Hispanics (U.S. Bureau of the Census, 2000). This population includes several ethnic groups: Japanese, Koreans, Filipinos, Vietnamese, and the largest group, Chinese. Each group maintains its own customs and traditions, and within each population these are likely to be more strongly adhered to by the first generation to immigrate.

Data on the health status of these populations are difficult to obtain due to the absence of any large national database and the lumping together of all of the populations into one group. Data from the American Heart Association show a high prevalence of diabetes, hypertension, and obesity among the older population, with heart disease and stroke the leading causes of death (American Heart Association, 2003). How-ever, data on the overall functional status or limitations of these popula-tions are lacking. Findings that are available tend to be on specific groups in one geographic area.

A study of Filipino, Indian, Japanese, Korean, and Vietnamese adults over age 65 in New York City found that on measures of general physical functioning, mental health, and social functioning, the group rated themselves lower than the general older population (Ryan, 2003). In addition, more than 40% reported depressive symptoms, making de-pression more prevalent than in the general elderly population. Poor mental health was most likely experienced when they felt a greater cultural gap between themselves and their children and were unable to read English. These limitations as well as their impairments in ADLs are associated with poorer social functioning.

NATIVE AMERICANS

The American Indian elderly are, according to many indices, the most impaired and potentially frail of any ethnic groups. The extent of this impairment is reflected by the fact that at age 45, American Indians experience limitations in their ADLs comparable to those experienced by other groups at age 65 (Cook, 1989). Older American Indians have a higher percentage than Whites of disabilities preventing them from using public transportation, with 71% having limitations in their ability to perform ADLs (Manson & Callaway, 1990).

Rates of chronic diseases such as heart disease, diabetes, and cancer are 600% higher for Native Americans than for the rest of the population (Office of Minority Health, 2002). Poor health education and health behaviors, poor facilities, and limited services are major causes of this ill health. As an example, one study found that hypertension was fre-quently not diagnosed or monitored, suggesting that improved mea-sures of detection and management were essential (Rhoades & Buchwald, 2003). Other research found that diabetes among the elderly contributed to poor role performance, health perception, and quality of life (McFall, Solomon, Teshia, & Smith, 2000). Education about the care of diabetes for both patients and their caregivers is needed in order to improve the management of the illness.

Data on the physical functioning of American Indian elders indicate that almost 25% rate themselves as disabled, with approximately 8% reporting more than one disability. In comparison to national data on limitations among the older population, Native Americans report increased limitations and needs for assistance at as young as age 55. At age 55, 30% need assistance with walking, in comparison to 11% of the general population age 65 and above (NRCNAA, 1998). It is also important to note that the same data indicate that only 6.5% of elders receive personal assistance to help with their limitations.

FAMILIES AND CAREGIVING

It is generally believed that family support networks among ethnic groups are strong and that they provide all the assistance a functionally impaired older relative may require. The fact that minority elderly are underrepresented in nursing homes is understood as evidence of a lack of need for such care and that families are providing for these persons in the community. Just as demographic changes are occurring with the majority population, however, parallel changes are occurring within the ethnic and minority populations.

Younger cohorts move from ethnic areas in inner cities, often leaving the older relatives to cope on their own or providing only minimal amounts of assistance. This lack of involvement can also increase feelings of stress and depression among older persons as they feel neglected and isolated by children who no longer respect them or adhere to traditional values and norms. If expectations not shared by adult children remain strong among the elderly, dissatisfaction can ensue regardless of the efforts that the children make.

Expectations for assistance are strongest among first generation immigrants and those not born in the United States. As younger cohorts become acculturated, traditional norms regarding caregiving may change along with the new norms and demands of society. Moreover, among many ethnic minority groups, the low economic status of adult children and other family members, as well as their own health problems, can make it extremely difficult to provide care to an impaired older person. At the same time, little is known about the extent to which family caregiving actually meets the needs of dependent seniors.

PREFERENCES FOR INFORMAL CARE

The degree to which a preference for informal care reflects traditional values and obligations, or previous negative experiences with the formal system, continues to be debated. Histories of discrimination, poor services, long waits, and culturally insensitive staffs can encourage a preference for and dependence on the family as a source of care. Moreover, in a period when immigrants are falling under increased scrutiny regarding their legal status, as well as their eligibility for some programs, the preference may indeed be for informal assistance rather than involvement with formal services.

A study of African American, Puerto Rican, and non-Hispanic Whites in an urban area found culture a more important factor than socioeconomic status in determining the amount of informal care. The two minority groups, regardless of income or disabilities level, received more informal care than older White persons (Tennstedt & Chang, 1998). Although these findings suggest a cultural preference for informal care, it is difficult to discern whether this preference reflects values and traditions, or negative attitudes and experiences with the formal system is undetermined.

Evidence for the salient role of ethnicity in the caregiving relationship is found in a study of first and second generation Japanese Americans living in Chicago. Filial piety, or support of the older generation, was a strong sentiment among both parents and their adult children (Osako & Liu, 1986). Adult children with more personal resources than their parents continued to accept the norms of filial responsibility, incorporating them into the pattern of American values that emphasize individual choice and independence. The tradition actually assisted in the older individual's transition from an independent to a dependent status.

Even among this population, though, the propensity for familial care may be waning. A study of Japanese American families in Washington State found that they were as interested in nursing home care as others in the population (McCormick et al., 1996). At the same time, a survey of supportive community services use by family caregivers in all groups of Asian Americans found only 15% using them, in comparison with approximately 30% of other caregivers (National Alliance for Caregiving, 1997). This lack of use may partially be explained by the finding that a larger proportion of Asian caregivers did not know what kind of help or information would be useful. Ensuring that educational materials and outreach tailored to specific ethnic groups are developed could foster the use of needed services.

The complexity of unraveling cultural factors from other determinants in the preference for informal care is vividly depicted in findings on Korean elderly. Low levels of service awareness and utilization of community long-term care services in comparison with non-Hispanic Whites were viewed as results of a lack of outreach and information (Moon, Lubben, & Villa, 1998). In addition, this underutilization may also indicate that services themselves are culturally inappropriate and persons are making conscious decisions not to use them (Cho, 1998).

INFORMAL SUPPORTS OF AFRICAN AMERICAN SENIORS

Much research has been done on the informal support systems of African American elderly, including the extent to which these systems are available to them. Older African Americans have been found to draw on a varied pool of informal helpers not restricted to immediate family, and in which there is some degree of substitution. When children are unavailable to assist the elderly, other relatives, particularly siblings, will provide care (Taylor, 1985).

This extended system increases the possibility of others to provide support. But kin and non-kin appear to play varying roles in meeting the needs of the elderly. Kin are found to provide long-term, instrumental assistance based on an obligatory relationship, while non-kin are more likely to provide socioemotional support and care for short-term needs (Taylor & Chatters, 1988). In comparison to White functionally impaired older persons, African Americans are more likely to have informal supports that are not members of the immediate family (Burton et al., 1995).

The type, amount, and frequency of help is on a sliding scale in these arrangements. Increases in disability contribute to increases in the number of available helpers and increased contacts, depending on the proximity of the family. However, the extent to which informal help to African American elderly is available should not be overestimated. The African American elderly are less likely to have spouses and adult children available to provide help and financial assistance.

In a study of the support systems of inner-city African Americans, Johnson and Baher (1990) found that adult children, even when close to the elderly, did not tend to offer instrumental support because of strains and distractions in their own lives. Moreover, older persons resisted being dependent on their children, preferring instead to use formal services such as home help and chore workers. Many with the most serious impairments had no weekly contact with either relatives and friends. Thus, those most in need of support may be the most at risk of being isolated due to their inability to maintain social networks.

The church has been viewed as a source of support for older African Americans, supplementing the social support offered by families (Taylor & Chatters, 1988; Walls & Zarit, 1991). However, research suggests that such assumptions may not be consistently valid. A study of frail urban African Americans found that they did not receive any more assistance than the non-frail from the church or from their families (Bowles et al., 2000). Contrary to assumptions regarding supports, the frail were less likely than others to feel close to their families and did not have greater contact with them. The group used more community services than others and did not report greater support from the church, indicating that the church was not involved in meeting their care needs. These findings reinforce the need to be cautious when assuming that needs of these older persons are being met without formal community help.

THE STRESS OF CAREGIVING

Ethnicity does not provide immunity from the stress of caregiving, although study results vary on how it relates to caregiver well-being. In a study of burden among Hispanic caregivers, Cox and Monk (1996) found that cultural values and norms continued to govern familial relationships and the care of the elderly. However, strong adherence to these values could have negative consequences on caregiver well-being. It may affect both their response to the use of services as well as the strains they experience. Among Hispanic caregivers, the use of formal services, although alleviating some of demands placed on the caregiver's time, was associated with greater depression. This finding suggests they felt troubled in not adhering to cultural expectations regarding caregiving (Cox & Monk, 1996).

Other studies on depression among Hispanic caregivers have looked at specific population subgroups. In one study Mexican American women reported significantly higher rates of depression than either Anglo or African American caregivers (Adams, Aranda, Kemp, & Takagi, 2002). Other research indicates Cuban caregivers are more depressed than non-Hispanic caregivers, with primary risk factors being female and caring for a relative with poor cognitive status (Harwood et al., 2000).

The impact of caregiving on the informal supports of African American elderly is noted in their care of relatives with Alzheimer's disease. A study of African American and White caregivers who had contacted Alzheimer's associations for assistance showed African American caregivers were not immune to the depression and strains experienced by their non-minority peers (Cox, 1999). However, their well-being was more strongly affected by the support they received from others than by the actual status of the patient. These caregivers maintained very strong expectations for assistance from other family members and when these expectations were not met, they became vulnerable to depression.

These findings imply that caution must be taken when attributing particular caregiver responses to specific groups. There may be as much diversity within groups as among individuals: Income, place of residence, relationship, employment, and degree of acculturation, as well as the degree of discrimination or racism experienced can have distinct influences on a caregiver's use of and response to formal services.

SERVICE USE

With the rates of disability and chronic illness among African American and Hispanic elderly higher than those of non-Hispanic Whites, and their use of institutional care lower, there is an implied need for community care and services. However, many factors can influence such use, including those associated with the individual and with the service itself. Understanding the influence of potential barriers impinging on the decision to use services is fundamental to assuring that specific needs are met.

Individual barriers are those associated with low income, a lack of insurance, inability to speak English or limited English, and immigration status. Persons who are insecure about their residency status and who are unable to understand program guidelines or criteria are particularly vulnerable to these barriers. In addition, individual barriers may refer to adherence to norms regarding the use of services. Thus, a person may be reluctant to use a support group for fear of stigma associated with sharing problems outside of the family. A family may choose not to use formal home care if the home attendants are from the same ethnic group and may judge them negatively for not providing all of the care themselves.

Services themselves can present barriers by not having ethnically diverse staff, lacking flexibility in their programs, and having little understanding of the groups they intend to serve. Without staff that can easily communicate with persons in their own language, interpreters, or materials that can be understood, programs risk being underutilized by ethnic populations. Users must also be assured the providers they see are as competent and qualified as those seen by other groups (Brach & Fraser, 2000). Locating services in ethnic neighborhoods and close to public transportation further contributes to utilization.

MODELS OF SERVICE UTILIZATION

The Andersen model of health services utilization (Andersen & Newman, 1973) is frequently used to provide a framework for examining the utilization of services by diverse groups. The model depicts utilization as resulting from three sets of factors: predisposing, enabling, and need. Predisposing factors are demographics and socioeconomic characteristics including race and ethnic background. Enabling factors can include economic resources, insurance, living environment, social resources, transportation, and personal resources. Needs encompass physical health, mental health, functional status, and one's own perception that services can help.

The model is often used to compare the use of in-home and community-based services by specific populations. However, in applying the model it is important to recognize that need itself, often a primary factor in determining service use, may be interpreted differently and thus is not necessarily a prerequisite for service use.

Cox (1999) applied the model to African American and White caregivers of Alzheimer's relatives. Both groups were comparable with regard to the needs of both patient and caregiver, and needs were motivating factors toward service use. Given this similarity, however, the groups differed in their interests in specific services. White caregivers were most interested in obtaining information on the illness and support groups, while the African American caregivers were more interested in day care, home health, referrals, and respite.

In a study applying the model to focus groups of White non-Hispanic and African American seniors, need played a less significant role than other factors in attitudes toward long-term care (Bradley et al., 2002). Predisposing and enabling factors such as attitudes and knowledge, social norms, and perceived control were most important in influencing service-use intention. Accessibility of information about long-term care, feelings toward the norms concerning caregiving, and concerns of privacy and self-determination were most important in predicting whether or not persons would use long-term care services.

Another model of service utilization (Wallace, 1990) views use as affected by structural factors associated with the availability, accessibility, and acceptability of services. Ethnic older adults and their families are at risk of finding barriers in each of these areas. Availability refers to the existence and provision of services. Accessibility involves eligibility criteria, insurance, and income as well as knowledge and awareness of services. Acceptability refers to the staff and the ways in which services are offered. If programs are made congruent with cultural values, recognizing attitudes toward the use of formal assistance, and concerns like fear of dependency by older persons, acceptability is increased.

The importance of acceptability of services is reflected in the use of services by Japanese Americans in Seattle (Young, McCormick, & Vitaliano, 2002). The Japanese community was involved in identifying the service needs of Japanese elders and in developing appropriate services such as a nursing home, assisted living, adult day care, and meal services. Accordingly, the services were developed in a way that made them culturally acceptable to both elders and their families. Care was taken to assure that the programs were perceived as an extension of traditional family caregiving. By incorporating attitudes and traditions of the population, the services were viewed positively and were well-utilized.

ON LOK

On Lok Senior Health Services in San Francisco is an example of how community care services can be developed to be accessible and acceptable to diverse populations of older adults. On Lok was established in 1971 in response to the health care needs of the frail elderly in San Francisco's Chinatown and surrounding areas. It began as a day care center for the elderly, and then served as a Medicare demonstration model of consolidated services providing all medical and social services.

On Lok has expanded into eight community sites in the San Francisco area. The population served by On Lok is primarily Asian or Pacific Islander (63%), as are the staff (74%) (Kornblatt, Eng, & Hansen, 2003). However, the program also serves large populations of Hispanic and Caucasian elderly. As program participants have become more diverse, a staff training program in cultural diversity has been introduced to increase knowledge about the specific cultures. The program was developed from the responses of staff to a survey that assessed their knowledge and understanding of the cultures of the various groups.

Based upon these responses, the following specific objectives for the training were developed:

1) Increase understanding of how culture determines attitudes, values, and behaviors;
2) Gain an overview of the dimensions of diversity that staff bring to the workplace;
3) Increase inter- and intra-cultural sensitivity toward both On Lok participants and staff;
4) Learn effective communication skills.

The training is seen as having contributed to both staff satisfaction and the quality of care they provide, with staff better able to understand and respond to the concerns and needs of participants.

REACHING DIVERSE GROUPS

One of the greatest challenges in meeting the care needs of ethnic elderly in the community is reaching them. For many reasons these persons, particularly those with the most needs, may be the most unconnected or suspicious of the service system. Overcoming the many barriers that can affect their use of services demands both knowledge and commitment by providers.

Working with persons from the community on plans for services development can be fundamental in assuring that programs are congruent with both the values and needs of the intended population. These persons are also important in helping to assure the credibility of the program and in communicating its aims. Including community residents on administrative boards can assist in developing valuable links with the community, crucial to its acceptability.

A key factor in assuring utilization is active outreach. Outreach involves more than having materials in different languages. It involves actively going into the community to develop relationships with groups and to inform them about the services, its intentions, and how it may meet the assistance needs of older persons and their families. Using workers from the same ethnic group as the intended client population can help increase the effectiveness of the outreach effort, as it can be easier for them to communicate and establish rapport. Language barriers affecting understanding of the problems of the older population are also reduced.

Outreach entails going to community fairs, churches, senior centers, physician offices, and other sites that older persons and their relatives may visit. These activities provide an opportunity to describe programs and respond immediately to questions and concerns. They are important in enabling providers to learn about factors affecting service utilization, and thus can help to assure that programs are congruent with the attitudes and expectations of the population.

Staff must be knowledgeable about traditions, norms, and values in order to interact effectively with a population. Through training and education, persons may learn about relevant cultures and become aware of their own biases and perspectives regarding specific groups. Such education can be as important for staff who share the same ethnicity as the clients as for other staff. As an example, if ethnic staff disapprove of a family's use of formal assistance, the attitudes can deter utilization. Thus ethnic group membership in itself is not sufficient to assure service use.

In designing services, it is essential that programs are presented in a manner sensitive to the cultural nuances of the population. Persons may be deterred from using services if they are confronted with many forms or must be interviewed by many different staff. Such procedures, often common in service agencies, can deter those who are used to more informal and intimate relationships. Collecting information needed for eligibility must be done in ways that are not perceived as intrusive or offending.

The ways programs present themselves can be important determinants in their acceptability. Many may be deterred from a program that focuses on mental illness or problems, while they would be accepting of one emphasizing growth and change. In the same way, relatives may respond more favorably to support services stressing the ways they can further enable them, rather than those that stress relief from the burdens of caregiving.

CULTURAL COMPETENCY

In recent years a growing recognition of the ethnic plurality of our society has occasioned increased interest in developing culturally competent professionals and services. Cultural competency has been defined as "a set of congruent behaviors, attitudes, and policies that come together in a system or agency or among professionals that permit them to work across cross-cultural situations" (National Association of Social Workers, 1997). Such competency may be viewed as a prerequisite for reaching and serving older ethnically diverse adults and their families.

Cultural competency demands that persons working with ethnic groups be knowledgeable about their values, beliefs, and traditions, and be respectful of them. Practitioners must be able to respond to these persons according to their preferences and their norms for behaviors. Communication is essential for cultural competency, and necessitates some fluency in the language and dialects of the persons being served. In addition, communication also implies understanding nonverbal gestures that persons use in their social interactions with each other and with those outside their ethnic groups. Sensitivity to this communication can be a critical factor in the group's acceptance of the provider and service.

Finally, cultural competency requires that practitioners be accepting of differences (Bhagat & Prien, 1996). Recognizing one's own biases and the ways they affect perceptions and expectations is fundamental to working effectively with culturally diverse older persons. Equally important is the avoidance of stereotyping, or assuming that all members of an ethnic group share the same beliefs and traditions. This is particularly important when working with older persons who may show much stronger adherence to traditional values and norms than their adult children.

SUMMARY

Ethnicity and culture are important influences on the aging process, caregiving, and even the responses of caregivers themselves. Relationships are consistently found between ethnicity and chronic disease as well as seniors' limitations and their responses to them. Such disparities occur even among subgroups of ethnic elderly. At the same time, it remains unclear the extent to which such variations are themselves the results of culture and traditions, or are reflections of continuing disparities resulting from histories of discrimination, poor access, inadequate care, and unresponsive services.

Families continue to play major roles in caring for older ethnic persons in the community and such care is often used to explain their relative lack of use of institutional care. However, many caregivers struggle to meet the demands of their older relatives and are not immune from many of the negative effects of caregiving. Both individual barriers and those presented by services can impact on utilization. Programs must to be sensitive and responsive to the needs of cultural groups, their values, and traditions, as well as their previous experiences with formal services. Service utilization depends upon careful planning, the involvement of community persons, well-trained staff, and effective outreach.

Cultural competency refers to the ability of persons to communicate and work effectively with persons from diverse backgrounds. It assumes specific training in cross-cultural work, as well as understanding of personal biases and beliefs that can affect interactions. An important aspect of cultural competency is the ability to accept the validity of differences and another person's values and perspectives.

Finally, it is essential to recognize that ethnicity is not a constant. Its influence on the life of an older person, and the ways he or she perceives impairments, assistance, and care will vary. Although ethnicity may be an important component in this process, it is not necessarily the only one. Seniors' experiences with formal services and past discrimination can be equally important determinants in the use and choice of care providers.

REFERENCES

Adams, B., Aranda, M., Kemp, B., & Takagi, K. (2002). Ethnic and gender differences in distress among Anglo American, African American, Japanese American, and Mexican American spousal caregivers of persons with dementia. *Journal of Clinical Geropsychology, 8,* 279–301.

American Heart Association. (2003). *Statistical fact sheet: Populations.* Author.

Andersen, R., & Newman, J. (1973). Societal and individual determinants of medical care utilization in the United States. *Milbank Quarterly, 51,* 95–124.

Becker, G., Beyee, B., Newsom, E., & Mayen, M. (2003). Creating continuity through mutual assistance: Intergenerational reciprocity in four ethnic groups. *Journal of Gerontology, Social Sciences, 58B,* S151–S159.

Benson, V., & Marano, M. (1998). Current estimates from the National Health Interview Survey, 1985–1994. In *Vital and Health Statistics* (Vol. 2, p. 110). Hyattsville, MD: National Center for Health Statistics.

Bhagat, R., & Prien, K. (1996). Cross-cultural training in organizational contexts. In D. Landis & R. Bhagat (Eds.), *Handbook of intercultural training* (2nd ed.). Thousand Oaks, CA: Sage.

Bowles, J., Brooks, T., Hayes-Reams, P., Butts, T., Myers, H., Allen, W., & Kington, R. (2000). Frailty, family, and church support among urban African American elderly. *Journal of Health Care for the Poor and Underserved, 11,* 87–99.

Brach, C., & Fraser, I. (2000). Can cultural competency reduce racial and ethnic health disparities: A review and conceptual model. *Medical Care Research and Review, 57,* 181–317.

Bradley, E., McGraw, S., Curry, L., Buckser, A., King, K., Kasl, S., & Andersen, R. (2002). Expanding the Andersen model: The role of psychosocial factors in long-term care use. *Health Services Research, 37,* 1221–1242.

Burnette, D., & Mui, A. (1995). In-home community-based service use by three groups of elderly Hispanics: A national perspective. *Social Work Research, 19*(4), 197–206.

Burton, L., Kasper, J., Shore, A., Cagney, K., LaViest, T., Cubbin, C., & German, P. (1995). The structure of informal care: Are there differences by race? *Gerontologist, 35,* 744–752.

Carrasquillo, O., Lantigua, R., & Shea, S. (2000). Differences in functional status of hispanic versus non-hispanic white elderly. *Journal of Health and Aging, 12,* 342–361.

Center for an Aging Society, Georgetown University. (2003). *Older Hispanic Americans: Less care for chronic conditions.* Washington, DC: Georgetown University.

Cho, P. (1998). Comment. *Gerontologist, 38,* 317–319.

Cox, C. (1995). Comparing the experiences of black and white caregivers of dementia patients. *Social Work, 40*, 343–349.

Cox, C. (1999). Service needs and use: A further look at the experiences of African American and White caregivers seeking Alzheimer's assistance. *American Journal of Alzheimer's Disease, 14*, 83–101.

Cox, C., & Monk, A. (1996). Strain among caregivers: Comparing the experiences of African American and Hispanic caregivers of Alzheimer's relatives. *International Journal of Aging and Human Development, 43*, 93–105.

Escalante, A., Barrett, J., del Rincon, I., Connnell, J., Phillips, C., & Katz, J. (2002). Disparity in total hip replacement affecting Hispanic Medicare beneficiaries. *Medical Care, 40*, 451–460.

Fritz, L., Ortiz, F., & Ponton, M. (2001). Frequency of Alzheimer's disease and other dementias in a community outreach sample of Hispanics. *Journal of the American Geriatrics Society, 49*, 1301–1308.

Gurland, B., Wilder, D., Lantigua, R., Mayeux, R., Stern, Y., Chen, J., & Killeffer, E. (1997). Differences in rates of dementia between ethnoracial groups. In L. Martin & B. Soldo (Eds.), *Racial and ethnic differences in the health of older Americans* (pp. 233–261). Washington, DC: National Academy Press.

Harwood, D., Barker, Ownby, R., Bravo, M., Aquero, H., & Duaro, R. (2000). Predictors of positive and negative appraisal among Cuban American caregivers of Alzheimer's disease patients. *International Journal of Geriatric Psychiatry, 15*, 481–487.

Institute of Medicine. (2002). *Unequal treatment: Confronting racial and ethnic disparities in healthcare.* Washington, DC: National Academy Press.

Johnson, C., & Baher, B. (1990). Families and networks among older inner city blacks. *Gerontologist, 30*, 726–733.

Johnson, J., & Smith, N. (2002). Health and social issues associated with racial, ethnic, and cultural disparities. *Generations, 26*, 25–32.

Kornblatt, S., Eng, C., & Hansen, J. (2003). Cultural awareness in health and social services: The experience of On Lok. *Generations, 26*, 46–53.

Lee, A., Gehlbach, S., Hosmer, D., Reti, M., & Baker, C. (1997). Medicare treatment differences for Blacks and Whites. *Medical Care, 35*, 1173–1190.

Manson, S., & Callaway, D. (1990). Health and aging among American Indians: Issues and challenges for the geriatric sciences. In M. Harper (Ed.), *Minority aging: Essential curricula content for selected health and allied health professions.* Health Resources and Services Administration, DHHS Pub. No. HRS (P-DV-90-4). Washington, DC: U.S. Government Printing Office.

Markides, K., Liang, J., & Jackson, J. (1990). Race, ethnicity, and aging: Conceptual and methodological issues. In L. George & R. Binstock (Eds.), *Handbook of the social sciences* (3rd ed.). New York: Academic Press.

Miller, B., Campbell, R., Davis, L., Furner, S., Giachello, A., Prohaska, T., Kaufman, J., Li, M., & Perez, C. (1996). Minority use of community long term care services: A comparative analysis. *Journal of Gerontology, Social Sciences, 51B*, S70–S81.

McFall, S., Solomon, T., Teshia, A., & Smith, D. (2000). Health related quality of Native American primary care patients. *Research on Aging, 22*, 692–714.

McCormick, W., Ohata, C., Uomoto, J., Young, H., Graves, A., & Kakull, W. (1996). Attitudes towards use of nursing homes and home care in elderly Japanese Americans. *Journal of the American Geriatrics Society, 50*, 1149–1155.

Moon, A., Lubben, J., & Villa, V. (1998). Awareness and utilization of community long-term care services by elderly Korean and non-Hispanic White Americans. *Gerontologist, 38*, 309–316.

Mui, A., & Burnette, D. (1994). Long term care service use by frail elders: Is ethnicity a factor? *Gerontologist, 34*, 190–198.

National Alliance for Caregiving. (1997). *Caregiver data for caregivers to the elderly 1987 and 1997*. Bethesda, MD: Author.

National Association of Social Workers. (1997). *Code of ethics*. Washington, DC: Author.

National Center for Health Statistics. (1999). *Health and aging chartbook*. Hyattsville, MD: Author.

Office of Minority Health. (2002). *National forum on health disparity issues for American Indians and Alaska Natives*. Denver: Author.

Osako, M., & Lui, W. (1986). Intergenerational relations and the aged among Japanese Americans. *Research on Aging, 8*, 128–155.

Rhoades, D., & Buchwald, D. (2003). Hypertension in older urban Native American primary care patients. *Journal of the American Geriatrics Society, 51*, 774–781.

Ryan, A. (2003). *Asian American elders in New York City: A study of health, social needs, quality of life, and quality of care*. New York: Asian American Federation of New York.

Shibutani, T., & Kwan, K. (1965). *Ethnic stratification*. New York: MacMillan.

Tang, M., Stern, Y., Marder, K., Bell, K., Gurland, B., Lagtigua, R., Andrews, H., Feng, L., Tycko, B., & Mayeux, R. (1998). The APOE-epsilon 4 allele and the risk of Alzheimer's disease among African Americans, Whites, and Hispanics. *Journal of the American Medical Association, 279*, 751–755.

Taylor, R. (1985). The extended family as a source of support to elderly Blacks. *Gerontologist, 25*, 488–495.

Taylor, R., & Chatters, L. L. (1988). Church members as a source of informal social support. *Review of Religious Research, 30*, 193–203.

Tennstedt, S., & Chang, B. (1998). The relative contribution of ethnicity versus socioeconomic status in explaining differences in disability and receipt of informal care. *Journal of Gerontology, Social Sciences, 53B*, S61–S70.

U.S. Bureau of the Census. (2000). *National population projections: NP-T4*. Washington, DC: U.S. Government Printing Office.

Wallace, S. (1990). The no-care zone: Availability, accessibility, and acceptability in community-based long term care. *Gerontologist, 30*, 254–262.

Wallace, S., Levy-Storms, L., Kingston, R., & Andersen, R. (1998). The persistence of race and ethnicity in the use of long term care. *Journal of Gerontology, Social Sciences, 53B*, S104–S112.

Walls, C., & Zarit, S. (1991). Informal support from black churches and the well-being of elderly blacks. *Gerontologist, 31*, 490–495.

White-Means, S. (2000). Racial patterns in disabled elderly persons' use of medical services. *Journal of Gerontology, Social Sciences, 55B*, S76–S89.

Young, H., McCormick, W., & Vitaliano, P. (2002). Attitudes toward community-based services among Japanese American families. *Gerontologist, 42*, 814–825.

Chapter 8

New Responses in Community Care

Enabling needy older persons to live and function as independently as possible in the community requires interventions on many levels. In many communities across the nation such interventions are occurring. Many are at the state level, focusing on persons who are already impaired and most often Medicaid-eligible. These programs tend to be designed to help maintain persons in their homes as long as possible, and thus delay the need for more costly institutionalization.

Through the use of home- and community-based service waivers (HCBS), states can offer an array of services to persons at home who would otherwise be in nursing homes. Medicaid also provides for personal care under a Personal Care Option in the state Medicaid plan. This means that such services can be provided to persons who meet the state's own criteria for personal care, which may differ from that of nursing home care.

States also develop separate state-funded programs for personal care that can permit them to provide for persons who are not Medicaid-eligible. These programs use general revenue funding as well as other state funds for the programs, and generally offer a wide array of services that may include emergency shelter, adult foster care, counseling, and training for informal caregivers. Some states provide home and community care services using several funding sources such as Medicaid, Older American funds, block grants, and other revenues. Overall program funding impacts on who is eligible to receive services and what programs are offered.

The importance to states of developing new systems of long-term care that do not rely on nursing homes is underscored by the National Governors Association. The association began a long-term care agenda in 2003 that includes involving government leaders, the business community, and citizens in a dialogue about preparing for an aging population. With Medicaid expenditures and the cost of nursing homes spiraling, long-term care has become a major concern. Among the issues the National Governors Association will focus on are identifying best practices that encourage community-based care, ways of supporting family caregivers, encouraging personal financial planning for health care, and conducting regional forums and workshops to identify innovative solutions (National Governors Association, 2003).

SOME STATE SYSTEMS OF CARE

Florida

Florida has developed a pilot project with managed long-term care in its Medicaid program, available in the Orlando and Palm Beach areas. The program includes incentives to HMOs for coordinating acute and long-term care services, using community-based programs as alternatives to more costly nursing homes.

In the pilot project, Long-Term Care Community Diversion Pilot Project, the state pays participating HMOs a capitated rate for all Medicaid services, including acute-care services not paid by Medicare, and home- and community-based services. The HMOs are responsible for unlimited nursing home payments, giving them strong incentives to reduce institutionalization as a means to reduce costs. Case managers employed by the HMOs coordinate acute- and long-term care services. They are also able to offer new benefits such as nutritional assessments, family training, and some financial help with assisted living costs that can help to reduce the need for nursing homes. These benefits are provided in addition to services that a person would be eligible for under Medicaid.

Enrollment in the project is voluntary and a participant can leave at the end of any month. At the same time, HMOs must accept any eligible applicant who wishes to enroll. Staff from the state assist with the application process when necessary. As part of the process, individuals receive a comprehensive assessment and review from the local Area Agency on Aging. Eligibility is restricted to persons 65 years of age and older, Medicaid- and Medicare-eligible, living in one of the pilot communities, and requiring a nursing-home level of care.

Within two weeks of enrollment, HMOs must conduct an in-person orientation with the enrollee, who receives a handbook describing all benefits, the roles of the case manager, and other information. The case manager develops an individual care plan, describing how the person will remain in the community. The managers consult with physicians, nurses, and pharmacists regarding appropriateness of medications and also coordinate medical appointments and arrange for the participant's transportation. Participants can appeal the decisions in the care plan or request a hearing.

During the fiscal year 2001 each HMO participating in the project received approximately $2,300 per month per person for all Medicaid benefits. This was higher than the payment for other Medicaid managed care programs, due to increased liability for nursing home costs and the program serving its maximum of 800 persons. Additional funding of the program in FY 2002–2003 has permitted the program to increase to 950 participants.

An evaluation of the program indicates that participants enrolled in the project report fewer unmet needs than those using the Medicaid waiver program (Florida Policy Exchange Center on Aging, 2001). Very few persons have decided to leave the program, with a disenrollment rate for HMOs of 2%–3% per month, mostly due to death or loss of Medicaid eligibility. The evaluation also found that participants in the project were less likely to live with an informal caregiver than those persons in waiver programs.

Minnesota

Minnesota integrates Medicare and Medicaid through its Minnesota Senior Health Options Program, in operation for 6 years. The program is open to all persons over the age of 65 who are eligible for Medicaid, but they do not need to be eligible for nursing home care, nor must they be assessed as eligible for nursing home care. However, enrollment is limited to those living in the 10 counties where the program is available. As of January 1, 2003, 4,875 persons were enrolled.

The program provides all home- and community-based services including assisted living, adult day care, home modifications, personal care attendants, and other services, as well as 180 days of nursing home care. Each participant has a care coordinator who may be employed by the health plan, clinic, or county and may be a nurse, social worker, or geriatric nurse practitioner. These persons are involved in all parts of the care from arranging services to monitoring them.

Three health plans have contracted with the state to integrate primary, acute, and long-term care services. Each plan must provide specific services such as risk screening and care coordination. The plans may also subcontract with other systems to coordinate services for participants. Medicare pays the plans directly, while Medicaid payments come from the state. For enrollees meeting criteria for nursing home admission but who continue to live in the community, the plans receive an increased payment or risk adjustment that is higher than the regular Medicare managed care payment. This adjustment makes it financially feasible to serve these persons in the community.

Among the reported accomplishments of the program are the following: reorganization of the service delivery system; development of geriatric care systems; reduced administrative duplication; one point of entry to primary, acute, and long-term care; low disenrollment rates; high satisfaction of enrollees and providers; increased access to home- and community-based services for underserved populations; and reduced rates of institutionalization.

The program is designed to provide flexibility and consumer direction while at the same time remaining financially practicable. It has also resulted in a geriatric care infrastructure that enables collaborations between health plans to develop new interventions. Because the state oversees the program, it stresses coordination as a model for providing quality health care for older persons in the community.

Oregon

Oregon is the first state to spend more on community-based care than on nursing homes, with more than 75% of Medicaid-eligible elderly receiving care in the home. In 1981 Oregon turned its long-term care system into the Senior and Disabled Services Division as a means of centralizing long-term care services through a system of centralized funding. The program sees nursing homes as the last resort for older persons, with all efforts made to maintain the person in the community. Long-term care funding through Medicaid is consolidated into one unitary budget. The size of the budget is determined by the legislature, which projects the numbers of persons who will be requiring services in various settings and gives provider rates for these settings.

There is a single entry point for all long-term care services, with a case manager creating individualized care plans. The managers are responsible for obtaining the funds from both public and private sources to give clients access to these services. Among the services are adult day care, respite, in-home services, adult foster care, residential treatment, and nursing home care. The state also offers caregiver training as well as increased assistance to caregivers. The single entry points themselves provide information on a multitude of services for older adults, ranging from health care to financial assistance and transportation. Both counseling and crisis intervention are also offered. For the majority of the state's population, Area Agencies on Aging (AAA) serve as the single entry points.

Case managers use laptop computers with an assessment instrument that immediately records responses and indicates what further information may be needed. The assessment details information on functioning, mental health status, physical health, resources, medications, and personal preferences. Certain responses indicate an immediate referral to a registered nurse so that a nursing home care plan can be developed.

Based upon the needs assessment, persons' assistance needs are ranked according to a 17-level priority scale. Whether or not assistance is given to persons at any specific priority level depends upon the program's budget. Until January 2003, persons in all 17 levels were given services. Eligibility has since been eliminated in levels 12–17, which include needing minimal assistance with mobility and eating, to needing full assistance with bathing or dressing. Approximately 4,800 persons, or 15% of those in the program, lost services.

Although cuts have occurred, the basic policy and structure of the program remain. Among the innovative features of the program are the coordination of institutional and community care into one long-term care agency, a single entry point for all services, a unitary services budget enabling care plans to be need-based, the establishment of priority levels for care, and the development of a quality management system.

Pennsylvania

The OPTIONS Program in Pennsylvania is available for all persons over the age of 60 having some degree of frailty in their physical or mental health status, or who are eligible for a nursing home. The program is administered through the Area Agencies on Aging and financed by funds from the Pennsylvania State lottery. Services include in-home services such as personal assistance, home support, short-term overnight respite, environmental modifications, counseling, transportation, and domiciliary care. Medicare, Medicaid, or a third-party payer cover home health services, which include home nursing. Consumer direction is a part of the program: Persons can choose to hire and supervise their own home-care attendant, or give the responsibility to the Area Agency on Aging.

Most persons receive care management with a manager assigned by the Area Agency on Aging. Together with the client, the manager designs a care plan that details services to be provided. The manager is responsible for ordering these services and monitoring the extent they meet the client's needs.

There are no financial eligibility criteria for OPTIONS, although beginning in 2002 cost-sharing was enacted. No sharing is required of persons with incomes below 125% of the poverty level. For persons above this level, the share will be calculated on their income and the cost of monthly services. If a person is Medicaid-eligible and the Area Agency on Aging has an opening for services through the Medicaid waiver, services will be provided through the waiver program.

Indiana

The Community and Home Options to Institutional Care for the Elderly and Disabled (CHOICE) program in Indiana is one part of the state's in-home services programming. CHOICE is funded through a variety of mechanisms including general state revenues, Older Americans Act funds, social services block grants, Medicaid, and private funding sources.

The State Bureau on Aging and In-home Services administers the program. The agency contracts with Area Agencies on Aging, which purchase services from local providers. Services range from case management to a variety of home-based services including respite care and day care. The services may also include transportation, adaptive equipment, and home modification.

The program is available to anyone with impairment in at least two ADLs; there is no income requirement. Pre-assessment screening is conducted by the Area Agency on Aging and is followed by a screening by a case manager. Working with the client, the manager develops a care plan. Informal care is incorporated into the plan with formal care provided by agencies with which the AAA has contracted. The case manager remains involved to monitor the care and the services. Fees for services are assessed on a sliding fee scale, with participants expected to cover part of the costs.

Nebraska

Nebraska's state legislature created the Nursing Facility Conversion Cash Fund in 1998. This program offered cash grants or low-cost loans to nursing homes to make transformations into assisted living or other type of less restrictive care facilities. The project permitted nursing home owners to incorporate these other types of care to maximize the cost-effectiveness of their services.

Owners had to reserve 40% of the newly constructed units for Medicaid-eligible persons, reduce licensed nursing home beds by at least the number of assisted living units created, and run the new facility for a minimum of 10 years. In addition, applicants had to provide a 20% match in funds that could be used for start-up costs, construction, training expenses, and first-year operating costs.

Over the course of the conversion program, which ended in 2001, $52.5 million was awarded to rural nursing homes for conversion. This resulted in 967 new assisted living units, 16 respite suites, and 27 adult day care programs. The program also resulted in savings to the state's Medicaid budget and a drop in nursing home occupancy (Coleman, Fox-Grage, & Folkemer, 2002).

New Jersey

New Jersey's Community Choice program was begun in 1998 as a program to provide nursing home residents and hospital patients with information about in-home services, housing alternatives, and community resources. The program is funded by state funds and grants from the Centers for Medicare and Medicaid Services.

Counselors and preadmission screening nurses are employed to help residents make decisions and assist them with transitions. Most persons making the transition to the community were older persons returning to their own homes or families, or moving into senior housing projects.

The program, in conjunction with inclusion of assisted living in the Medicaid waiver, has resulted in a slight decline of Medicaid nursing home residents. Such a decline could net savings in the overall Medicaid budget, as community care and assisted living cost less than nursing home care.

An evaluation of the program by Rutgers University finds participants pleased with it, reporting high satisfaction with their living arrangements. Ninety-three percent reported that the new situation was better than being in a nursing home (Howell-White, 2003). Persons felt that their quality of life had improved, and even if they had unmet needs they did not feel their ability to remain in the community was jeopardized. The federal government is aware of the need to further encourage states to develop community care services for persons with disabilities, and to use these services to replace nursing home care.

FEDERAL INITIATIVES

A new program, "Money Follows the Individual Rebalancing Demonstration," has been proposed by the government. The program would allot $350 million dollars to the states in FY 2004 to assist them in developing their long-term care systems to accomplish more effective choices between institutional and community care. Medicaid money would be available for those making the transition from institutions to the community and federal funds would cover the full cost of home- and community-based waiver services for one year. After that period, states would be responsible for continuing the care under their Medicaid budgets.

The program gives states the ability to design their own innovative programs offering older adults with impairment further choice in their decision of where to live. As funds are redistributed to the community, they will ideally also save states the costs of more expensive institutional care.

In 2001, the Center for Medicare and Medicaid Services (CMS) began implementing the Systems Change Grants for Community Living program. The goals of the program are to permit individuals a) to live in the least restricted environments, with necessary supports and in accordance with their individual preferences; b) exercise meaningful choices about their living environments, their service providers, the types of supports they use, and the manner by which services are provided; c) obtain quality services in a manner as consistent as possible with their community-living preferences and priorities.

Four types of grants are available: nursing home transition grants to assist states in helping persons transition from nursing homes to the community; community-integrated personal assistance and support grants to improve consumer direction and control over services; real choice system change grants to permit states to develop new community support systems; and technical assistance grants to communities. Since 2001, 48 grants totaling $125 million have been awarded to states.

Rhode Island is using its grant to hire service coordinators to assist with transitional activities from nursing homes and for support for referrals and communication. Nebraska is using its funds to develop a communication and marketing campaign to enhance public awareness of alternatives to nursing homes. In addition, the project is enlisting Area Agencies on Aging and trained ombudsmen to help identify and support nursing home residents who could move to the community. Both Alaska and North Carolina are using the grants to help develop consumer-directed programs, giving seniors more control over their personal budgets.

The Administration on Aging and CMS initiated grants in 2003 for states to develop Aging and Disability Resource Centers. The centers will offer one-stop entry points into long-term care systems and also serve as resources for professionals. The centers are a part of the New Freedom Initiative, working toward overcoming barriers to community care. States will be able to use the funds to redesign or better coordinate their systems of long-term care access, information, and assistance.

FEDERAL DEMONSTRATIONS FOR INTEGRATED CARE

Program of All-Inclusive Care for the Elderly (PACE)

The Program of All-Inclusive Care for the Elderly (PACE) was authorized by the Balanced Budget Act of 1997 as a system for developing comprehensive services, both acute and long-term, using both Medicare and Medicaid funding. The focus is on enabling persons over the age of 55 years, who would otherwise be institutionalized, to continue living at home. There are 24 PACE demonstration programs in the country and 2 permanent ones.

The providers receive monthly Medicare and Medicaid payments (if the person is Medicaid-eligible) for each enrollee. If the person is not Medicaid–eligible, he or she is responsible for paying the Medicaid portion of the premium, and Medicare covers the remainder. There is no limitation to the number, amount, or duration of services that a person can receive. Prescription drugs and transportation to the program and for required services are covered in the plan.

An interdisciplinary team assesses participant needs and develops individualized care plans. All services are provided through the PACE program, including social and medical services, day health, and in-home care. The goal of the plan is to maintain the person in the community but if a nursing home placement becomes necessary, PACE will pay for the care and the person will continue to be supervised by the PACE team.

Evaluations of these programs should help to indicate the specific services most needed and those who can best benefit from them. Such information can be used to increase effectiveness and to help implement the programs throughout the country.

Social Health Maintenance Programs (SHMOs)

The Centers for Medicare and Medicaid Services (CMS) have funded a demonstration project called Social Health Maintenance Organizations

(SHMOs), that integrates acute and long-term care for Medicare beneficiaries. Currently there are four SHMOs in operation, located in Portland, Oregon; Long Beach, California; Brooklyn, New York; and Las Vegas, Nevada. The plans offer similar services but have varying premiums and copayments.

Among the long-term care services they offer are care coordination, prescription drugs, short-term nursing home care, homemakers, personal care services, adult day care, and medical transportations. Some plans also include hearing aids, eyeglasses, and dental benefits. Participants' needs for services are assessed at enrollment and every 12 months.

An evaluation of the plans found no consistent evidence that participants were more likely to use skilled nursing homes and home health care than those outside of the plan (Thompson, 2002). There was also no evidence that the quality of care they received was better than that of other Medicare beneficiaries. Overall, the findings indicated that beneficiaries did not have better health outcomes than did persons in traditional Medicare, suggesting the SHMOs model is not effective. As noted in the evaluation, however, the lack of significant findings may have been affected by the fact that the study was too short in duration to demonstrate positive effects and because services were directed at a broad population rather than those who could have benefited most. Based on the findings and the higher costs generated by SHMOs, CMS has recommended that SHMOs be transitioned into standard Medicare +Choice plans.

Long-Term Care Partnership Programs

Four states, California, Connecticut, New York, and Indiana, offer a partnership program between state governments and private long-term care insurers. The purpose of these partnership programs is to provide access to affordable private long-term care insurance to moderate-income persons not able to afford private insurance coverage. They are permitted to get help from Medicaid without becoming impoverished.

Legislation introduced into Congress in 2003 would permit more states to enter into these partnerships. Presently, expansion of the program is restricted due to policies requiring new partnership states to recover assets from beneficiaries on their death. Because this requirement affects the family, it acts as a barrier to participation.

Persons who purchase the policies are insured for covered long-term care expenses for a predetermined level of benefits, through a private insurer. If the benefits under the private plan are exhausted and services are still needed, Medicaid is available, but in comparison to other Medicaid eligibility requirements, there is no requirement to spend down all assets to qualify. The purchasers are permitted to retain assets equal to the amount of benefits purchased under the policy. Medicaid becomes the payer only after the long-term care partnership benefits are exhausted.

The program represents an effort to integrate public and private sectors in long-term care protection. With states anxious to confront the rising costs of long-term care services, the National Governors Association supports the revised legislation that will make the program more attractive to consumers.

Private Initiatives

The Robert Wood Johnson Foundation (RWJF) is funding a $20 million initiative, Community Partnerships for Older Adults, to assist communities in improving their systems for delivering long-term care and supportive services to vulnerable older persons and their caregivers (RWJF, 2002). The program offers grant awards and technical assistance to projects that involve collaboration between business, community agencies, consumers, and government.

It is anticipated that 30 sites will be selected over an 8-year period for either development or implementation grants. The initiative focuses on three aims:

1) Mobilize communities to become involved in long-term care by increasing awareness of the roles and needs of older persons, educating persons to become better long-term care consumers, and strengthening community partnerships.
2) Improve access to services through better communication, increased coordination of services, and the leveraging of public and private resources.
3) Promote a better lifestyle for older persons by enhancing choices and decision making, and responding to diverse needs of caregivers.

WORKFORCE ISSUES AND RESPONSES

The quality of care received by older adults is dependent upon a skilled, knowledgeable, and caring workforce. Efforts to address these concerns are occurring at several levels with projects being initiated by both government and private foundations.

In addition to the design and structure of programs that can assist persons to remain in the community, there are major concerns about the shortage of a qualified, skilled workforce to care for this population. Professionals trained and educated in geriatric care (e.g., physicians, nurses, social workers) are critical for providing the types of care that older persons require. There is also a shortage of direct service providers, nurses aides, and other paraprofessionals, who play major roles in facilitating the ability of older persons to remain in their homes. The lack of a trained workforce has been described as the biggest problem in long-term care policy (Stone, 2000).

The need for physicians is vividly depicted in the comparison of geriatricians with pediatricians. In 2000, there were 62,386 pediatricians to treat 59 million children up to the age of 14, or one physician for every 945 children. This is contrasted with 9,000 geriatricians to treat 35 million persons 65 years and older, or one physician for every 3,888 persons (Alliance for Aging Research, 2002).

Federal policy makers are beginning to recognize the need for geriatric training, and provided increased funding for geriatric programs operated by the Health Resources and Services Administration (HRSA) in 2003. In 2004 $4.7 million in Geriatric Academic Career Awards was appropriated to encourage the development of academic geriatricians in medical schools.

One of the most pressing problems is the shortage of nurses aides and nursing assistants in both nursing homes and home-care agencies. In home-care agencies, jobs for nurses aides are expected to increase by 58% between the years 1998 and 2008 (Government Accounting Office [GAO], 2001). Yet the dearth of workers to fill these positions remains a challenge.

Not only is there a shortage of these workers, there are major problems in retention, with turnover rates of home-care aides of 28% in 2000 (American Health Care Association, 2003). Discouragement over poor work environments, low wages, and few benefits, and poor teamwork or peer support for learning are among the reasons attributed to this high turnover rate. Retention has also been found to be associated with adequacy of training, methods of workload management, career advancement, respect from administrators, organizational recognition, workloads and staffing levels, clarity of roles, and participation in decision making.

The rate of workplace injuries among nurses aides is alarmingly high—13 per 100 employees in 1999, a rate that surpassed that of the construction industry's 8 per 100 employees (GAO, 2001). At the same time, it is particularly troubling that many workers cannot afford health insurance either for themselves or their families. Salaries remain very low with home-care aides earning even less than those in nursing homes ($12,265 per year compared with $13,285 for those in institutions). Home-care aides are also less likely to have benefits, employer's health insurance, or pensions.

According to the GAO report (2001) most states have developed some initiatives to begin to deal with the severe shortage of direct service workers in both nursing homes and home care agencies. These initiatives are categorized as those dealing with wages and benefits, training and opportunities for advancement, and additional employee supports including better work environments, job skills, and social supports. Evaluations of these programs and their effects on the workforce are being conducted, but at present it is impossible to know how they will affect either turnover or retention, or the quality of care provided. Additionally, a federal policy establishing wages and benefits for these workers is not likely in a period of declining budgets.

Mental Health

The need for mental health care among older persons is indicated by a prevalence rate for psychiatric disorders, not including dementia, of 13% (Bartels & Smyer, 2002). It is estimated that the number of older persons with mental illness requiring care will continue to increase, with 15 million older adults having a mental illness in 2030 (Jeste, 1999). There remain serious concerns regarding the inadequate supply of professionals to meet the mental health needs of this population. Few persons receive specialized training in either geriatric psychiatry or psychology. Reflective of this is the fact that only 30% of accredited psychology programs offer any elective course in aging and only 10% offer a geriatric emphasis in their doctoral programs (Halpain, 1999).

Although social workers could play major roles in meeting the mental health and social needs of older persons, very few are attracted to geriatric care. As with the other mental health professions, only approximately 5% describe aging as their primary practice (Rosen & Zlotnik, 2001). However, efforts are under way, primarily through the private sector, to encourage more students to focus on gerontology.

The John A. Hartford Foundation has begun a program funding the development of geriatric curricula in schools of social work and supporting faculty interested in aging. The foundation also supports a partnership program that connects communities and practitioners through internships. One of the aims of the foundation is to assure that all social-work students receive some content in aging during their studies, even if they do not specialize in gerontology. The Hartford Foundation is also supporting geriatric training in nursing and medical programs.

Social workers and other health care professionals working in teams are also supported by the Department of Veterans Affairs through the Geriatric Education and Clinical Center (GRECC) program. Geriatric Education Centers (GECs) supported by the Health Resources Services Administration focus on the professional development of persons, educators, and practitioners working with older persons. As of 2003, 35 GECs have been funded across the country, focusing on multidisciplinary education and initiatives to meet the needs of the aging population.

An area that remains troubling is that of geriatric case management. For many older persons in the community, case managers are depended upon to assess needs, develop care plans, monitor progress, and act as advocates. However, although credentials are available for case managers, they are not required. Consequently, without stringent licensing requirements in states, persons calling themselves geriatric case managers may have had no more experience than caring for an elderly relative. This lack of any specific training or skills is particularly troubling when there are no immediate relatives living near the older person, fostering complete reliance on the manager.

As universal certification and licensing requirements are not forthcoming, it is critical for the public to be informed and knowledgeable about the backgrounds of geriatric case managers. At minimum, they should be knowledgeable about the educational background of the manager, years of supervision in client services, and experience in working with older persons.

Paraprofessionals

The federal government, states, and private foundations have become aware of the potential crisis among paraprofessional workers and have begun several projects, as well as passing legislation, to deal with it. The National Initiative on Paraprofessional Long-Term Care Workers has been implemented by the Department of Health and Human Services in partnership with the Paraprofessional Healthcare Institute to address both the shortage and retention of qualified workers.

The purposes of the initiative are as follows:

Increase public recognition of the role played by these workers.

Promote innovation at the state, community, and provider levels to improve recruitment and retention.

Create a national clearinghouse database on the long-term care workforce.

Increase understanding of the causes of the shortage so that policies, programs, and practices can be implemented to resolve them.

Collaborate with potential funders to plan and implement a program of applied research, demonstration, and evaluation to improve recruitment and retention.

The initiative will also develop a "tool kit" for states and providers for assessing effectiveness of workforce improvement policies and practices.

The Centers for Medicare and Medicaid (CMS) plan on funding several programs that also test solutions for the shortage of direct service workers in the community. Based upon findings from a survey of paraprofessionals conducted under the new Freedom Initiative, $6 million was allocated in FY 2003 for projects that might impact on the recruitment and retention of the workforce. The projects must focus on the provision of health insurance benefits, career ladders, continued education, time off for workers, wellness programs, and cultural competency development.

Using money from the Health Care Reform Act of 2000, New York City received 28 million dollars from the state to improve their health care coverage in 70 home care and personal care agencies. Evaluations are being conducted to determine whether these increased benefits can contribute to a more stable workforce by reducing agency turnover.

Washington State passed legislation in 2001 permitting home-care workers to unionize and bargain collectively with the state. The measure creates the Home Care Quality Authority, which oversees the recruitment, training, and standards for home-care workers who contract with the state. The authority also acts as a clearinghouse to connect workers with clients for hiring. The union acts as a bargaining agent with the state for wages as well as for benefits and insurance.

In 2000, Oregon also allowed home-care workers the right to organize and participate in collective bargaining. Workers are not direct state employees but work under contract to provide services. With the new contract, workers receive a salary increase, health benefits, workers' compensation, and paid leave. Under the contract, a board has also been created to provide training and to keep a registry for clients to enable them to find workers.

Unions may offer home-care workers a means of ensuring higher salaries and benefits; however, it is not clear they will be adequate in addressing concerns regarding effective recruitment and retention of home-care workers. Even with unionization, salaries remain low and state budgets are not in positions to greatly increase them. Moreover, it is unclear whether unionization can deal with many other problems, such as a lack of a career ladder and job-associated demands, so that work in this field actually becomes more attractive to workers.

Private foundations have also become involved in programs aimed at the recruitment and retention of direct-care workers. Better Jobs/ Better Care is a demonstration program funded by the Robert Wood Johnson Foundation and the Atlantic Philanthropies. The grants to states are for development and implementation of policy changes and practice interventions addressing the workforce shortage and the quality of direct-care providers' jobs, at state and local levels. The grants are expected to indicate best practices for attracting persons, reducing high turnover rates, and improving workforce quality.

There are four areas in which grants will be given: federal and state long-term care policy interventions; the organization, management and culture of the workplace; job preparation and ongoing education and training of direct-care workers; and approaches to expanding the pool of available workers.

HOUSING

Basic to addressing the needs of older persons in the community is adequate and appropriate housing. According to findings from the Commission on Affordable Housing and Health Facility Needs for Seniors in the 21st Century, presented to Congress in 2002, there remains a crisis due to a lack of affordable housing for older persons. Federal funding fails to keep pace with increased needs for alternative housing (alternative to institutions) for persons with physical and cognitive impairments. Among the commission's recommendations were preservation and renovation of existing housing, expanding successful housing productions, rental assistance programs, home- and community-based services, and supportive housing; linking shelter and services to promote and encourage aging in place; reformation of federal financing programs; and creation of new housing and service programs, models, and demonstrations.

One effort of the federal government in response to this need for suitable housing is a program through the Department of Housing and Urban Development (HUD), named Multifamily Housing Service Coordinator Grants. The grants have been given to owners of private housing developments in 42 states who receive HUD money for low-income persons. The grants are for hiring service coordinators who will assist frail older persons and those with disabilities to get services. The coordinators must have backgrounds in the social services.

Innovations and developments in senior housing that may reduce dependency on institutional care are occurring at the state and local levels. Iowa's Coming Home Project, sponsored by a grant from the Robert Wood Johnson Foundation to develop affordable assisted living, particularly in rural areas, has worked toward simplifying the development of these projects by assisting developers and service providers. With this technical assistance, the number of assisted-living homes increased from 16 to 46 in 2002. The first project had 54 units for low-income elderly and persons with disabilities and currently maintains a waiting list. A home care agency and the local Area Agency on Aging provide support services. The project is expected to save $800,000 annually in federal and state funds (Iowa Finance Authority, 2003).

The Coming Home Project is also using money from the Department of Housing and Urban Development to convert 22 units in a housing complex to assisted-living quarters, which will have a resident service coordinator. A second grant from the USDA Rural Community Development Initiative is being used to produce affordable assisted living through both new construction and conversion.

The Seattle Housing Authority has developed a housing community for low-income older persons using funds from Section 202, the Low Income Housing Credit, and non-profit groups. The housing includes 318 units in three buildings, and a large community area. One building will stress coordination of services by having a manager who can assist residents obtain services. This building operates under Section 202 housing, so that rents are equivalent to 30% of the tenants' incomes.

A second building has 84 studio- and one- and two-bedroom apartments, all wheelchair accessible. This building is for persons 62 years and older whose income is no more than 60% of the median gross income for the region. A third building has 154 assisted-living units. Located in the center of the complex are a computer room, dining room, shop, offices, and a fitness room. The complex is also adjacent to a park and close to shops and public transit.

The Miami-Dade Housing Authority converted an underutilized independent living complex into assisted-living units, being the first in the country to offer assisted living to elderly public housing residents (Department of Housing and Urban Development, 2001). The project was developed by linking, through the Medicaid waiver, low-income housing subsidies with Medicaid funding. Presently, HUD pays for housing expenses while Medicaid funds meals, services, and transportation. The housing authority has a case manager on site who assesses residents and reports directly to the authority, while a consulting firm manages the buildings. The complex provides multiple levels of services to meet diverse and changing needs of the residents. According to research from the housing authority, the per-capita long-term care costs may be as little as one quarter of those of a nursing home.

SUPPORT FOR FAMILY CAREGIVERS

With families the primary supports of older persons in the community, programs to support and relieve them are urgently needed. The primary support from the federal government comes through the National Family Caregivers Support Act (NFSCA), that permits states to use funds for several types of programs. A study from the Family Caregivers Alliance reports on programs initiated under the act in ten states. Although new programs continue to be created, this initial report, based on interviews with state officials and program representatives in each of the states, offers some idea of the ways the grant is being implemented and the challenges states continue to face (Family Caregivers Alliance, 2002).

Respondents were divided with regard to the recognition given to family caregivers. While most state officials believed they were generally recognized in state long-term care services, those involved with caregivers through organizations such as the Alzheimer's Association, Area Agencies on Aging, and other resource centers, generally felt there was not sufficient caregiver recognition or support. In addition, the term "caregiver" does not have a consistent meaning since in some states it applies only to paid caregivers and not family members.

This confusion is also apparent with regard to identifying the client. Disparities arose over whether it was the family, the informal caregiver, or the care recipient. Nearly half of state officials saw the older person as the client, less than one quarter felt it was the caregiver, and just over one quarter believed it was the family. In states initiating caregiver programs with NDCSA funds, the view of a family caregiver as a consumer or client was a new concept. Persons representing programs and agencies dealing with caregivers were consistent in identifying the family as the client.

States that had existing caregiver programs, such as Pennsylvania and Washington, used the new funds to augment these programs by broadening eligibility and expanding services. California, which also had a caregiver program, used the money to provide caregiver support to those caring for persons with cognitive impairment. Georgia used the funds to expand its voucher program for caregivers for their purchase of services from approved providers. States also differ in the extent to which caregiver support programs are integrated into other long-term care programs, with some having it an isolated program and others having it a part of their home- and community-based services.

According to the findings, caregivers need a multitude of services and options with the greatest needs being for respite care, assistive devices, consumable supplies, and home modifications. Although the funds were helpful, in most of the 10 states there were regional variations in access to services. Difficulties stemmed from efforts to balance an AAA's flexibility in developing service options and meeting statewide standards and uniformity with regard to support services. However, the overall trend was to give the AAAs more options, with the result being inconsistent services.

Several issues emerge from this preliminary study of the implementation of the NFCSA. There must be more federal- and state-level policy attention given to a family systems approach, with more support to the family and informal caregivers. The present level of funding is inadequate for real systems change, since many gaps in services remain. There also needs to be coordination of caregiver support services at all levels to reduce fragmentation and to assure that persons do have service options.

Another federal initiative through the Administration on Aging is the Eldercare Locator. This is a toll-free phone service that can also be accessed through the Internet. It gives families information and referrals to local services. The program provides assistance with legal, financial, and health care issues, and offers materials to assist adult children in discussing issues such as living arrangements with their parents. The majority of information requests regards home assistance, with half of the calls received coming from the older person rather than a family caregiver.

Other Initiatives

The Robert Wood Johnson Foundation provides grants under an initiative called Faith in Action. This program helps communities organize groups of volunteers from religious congregations and other community organizations to assist older persons with chronic health problems. They offer a range of services such as grocery shopping, errands, friendly visiting, and help paying bills. Over 1,000 volunteer programs have been created since the program began in 1984. The foundation continues to support the program, with over $75 million committed to it.

The Rosalynn Carter Institute for Human Development was begun in 1997 and focuses on all aspects of caregiving. The institute provides funds for research, education, and training that can support the well-being of caregivers. The Institute is also involved in advocacy and policy development, and disperses information about best practices in caregiving.

Finally, there are several associations and Internet sites focusing on the needs of family caregivers. Many of these associations are involved in advocacy and research activities as well. Assistance is provided on-line as well as through educational materials and brochures. The Alzheimer's Association has developed extensive services and resources for family caregivers ranging from information to support groups, respite care, and case management.

Technology

The use of technology to assist older persons in the community takes many forms. In some states, both the State Units on Aging and the Area Agencies on Aging are developing computer-based systems to assist with case management and the tracking of clients. The systems are also used for information, referral, and record keeping. Computer-based systems have also been developed that can assess persons' eligibility for benefits as well as provide referrals to appropriate services.

Technology is also being developed to make the home environments of older persons more appropriate to their needs. As well as independent projects developed through corporations and research facilities, the Administration on Aging, in conjunction with the National Center for Senior Housing Research, provides grants to pilot projects developing assistive technology and aging-in-place demonstration programs. The aim of this program is to increase public awareness of the needs of older persons and the possibilities of assistive technology. The grants will be used to demonstrate and implement new models that can be replicated and can contribute to independence of older persons and the well-being of their caregivers.

SUMMARY

Efforts are occurring in many spheres to redefine and reshape the long-term care system and its services so that older persons at risk of being institutionalized can be better able to remain in the community. Even with state budgets in precarious positions, many programs are being initiated that work toward increased linkage and coordination of services and their integration. Private foundations are playing key roles in the support of many of these innovations, both independently and in conjunction with publicly funded agencies. Moreover, this type of collaboration is itself conducive to the formulation of innovative practices that can serve older persons in the community.

Equally important is the focus being given to the workforce—both professional and nonprofessional—that provides care for this older population. Federal, state, and private funding has been made available for projects that examine recruitment and retention strategies. As the results from these efforts become known, it will be imperative to disperse them so that strategies and practices may be more widely adapted.

REFERENCES

Alliance for Aging Research. (2002). *Medical never-never land: 10 reasons why America is not ready for the coming age boom.* Washington, DC: Author.

AARP. (2003). *Beyond 2003: A report to the nation on independent living and disability.* Washington, DC: Author

American Health Care Association. (2003). *Results of the 2002 AHCA survey of nursing staff vacancy and turnover in nursing homes.* Washington, DC: Author.

Bartels, S., & Smyer, M. (2002). Mental disorders of aging: An emerging public health crisis. *Generations, 26,* 14–20.

Coleman, B., Fox-Grage, & Folkemer, D. (2002). *State long term care: Recent development and policy directions, 2003 update.* Washington, DC: National Conference of State Legislatures.

Family Caregivers Alliance. (2002). *Family caregiver support: Policies, perceptions, and practices in ten states since the passage of the National Family Caregiver Support Program.* San Francisco: Author.

Florida Policy Exchange Center on Aging. (2001). *Preliminary evaluation of Medicaid waiver managed long-term care diversion programs: Final report.* Tampa, FL: Author.

Government Accounting Agency. (2001). *Nursing workforce: Recruitment and retention of nurses and nurses aides is a growing concern,* (GAO-01-750T). Washington, DC: U.S. Government Printing Office.

Halpain, M. (1999). Training in geriatric mental health: Needs and strategies. *Psychiatric Services, 50,* 1205–1208.

Housing and Urban Development (HUD). (2001, Jan./Feb.). Miami Housing Agency brings assisted living to frail elderly. In *FieldWorks*. Washington, DC: Author.

Howell-White, S. (2003). *Current living situation and service needs of former nursing home residents: An evaluation of New Jersey's nursing Home Transition Program.* Rutgers Center for State Health Policy. New Brunswick, NJ: RCSHP.

Iowa Finance Authority. (2003). *Iowa Coming Home Project, special housing needs.* Author.

Jeste, D. (1999). Consensus statement on the upcoming crisis in geriatric mental health. *Archives of General Psychiatry, 56*, 848–853.

National Governors Association. (2003). *A lifetime of heath and dignity: Confronting long term care challenges in America.* Downloaded April 1, 2004, from http://www.nga.org/chairman03

Robert Wood Johnson Foundation. (2002). *Community partnerships for older adults.* Downloaded April 1, 2004, from http://rtjf.org

Rosen, A., & Zlotnik, J. (2001). Social work's response to the growing population. *Generations, 25*, 69–71.

Stone, R. (2000). *Long-term care for the elderly with disabilities: Current policy, emerging trends, and implications for the twenty-first century.* New York: Milbank Memorial Fund.

Thompson, T. G. (2002). *Report to Congress on evaluation results for the Social/Health Maintenance Organization II Demonstration.* Washington, DC: Department of Health and Human Services.

Chapter 9

The Challenges of Caring
for an Aging Society

As the century continues to mature, its residents will continue to place new demands on policies and services. The aging of the population will continue to challenge institutions to provide new and creative responses. Assuring that persons have adequate incomes, health care, and living arrangements to enable them to continue living in the community are among the greatest challenges. Moreover, assuring persons options about where and how to live their lives and about the care they receive is a particularly formidable task. The importance of self-determination and control cannot be underestimated. To the extent that care subordinates or suppresses autonomy, its benefits come at a dubiously high cost of human individuality and freedom (Collopy, 1988).

In addressing these challenges, it is essential to formulate responses from a very broad perspective. The needs of older persons cannot be subsumed under a single system or relegated to only one setting. For instance, good health and functioning in old age are not dependent solely upon the medical system. A secure and sound income, a stable support system, appropriate housing, and transportation are equally essential to assure the autonomy and dignity of older people.

An aging society demands comprehensive and consistent policies, services, and supports. On the federal level, the Administration on Aging and the Older Americans Act offer a foundation for the development of responsive policies. However, their ability to effectively meet the needs of the older population is challenged by limited resources. Services such as home repair and modifications, home attendants, and respite care will continue to be in short supply until a real commitment to aging and home- and community-based care is made.

As a result of multiple funding streams, service delivery systems, and subsequent eligibility requirements, community care remains fragmented, and older persons and their families needing assistance remain at risk. Although some steps, such as development of single entry points to care and case management, are being used to rectify the gaps that exist, they are not universally accessible. Making sure persons are knowledgeable about services are linked to them, and that these programs are effective in meeting their needs are essential for viable community care.

In addition, as programs develop, it is critical to recognize that options for care are crucial. As persons' needs, status, and desires vary, so may their interest in any particular program. Thus, whereas day care or case management may be appealing to some, others may feel more comfortable with assistance in the home or organizing their own services. Having options for care must be a right rather than a privilege if dignity and autonomy are to be sustained.

Many states use the Medicaid waiver to expand the array of home-based and community care services. However, the capacity of this program to meet the needs of seniors is strictly limited by its budgets and eligibility requirements, which focus on those with the lowest incomes and often those at risk for nursing home placement. Consequently, many of the innovative programs being developed under the waivers are not available to many older persons.

To date, our responses to the care of older persons in the community have been neither coordinated nor comprehensive. Developments in housing are not necessarily matched with equal developments in transportation or health care. Programs are not universally available or accessible. This results in options for care remaining closely linked with individual resources. Until the government sees aging and the community care needs of older persons as major issues to confront, the resources necessary to develop a viable and significant community care system will be lacking. Community care will continue to be the prerogative of those having the ability to pay or those "fortunate" enough to receive services under the Medicaid waiver. The vast majority of older Americans requiring assistance will continue to struggle to find appropriate and affordable services.

As long as Medicaid's bias toward institutions as the primary places for receiving assistance continues, a commitment to community care for older persons remains in jeopardy. The total spending for long-term care by Medicaid in 2000 was 72.5% for institutional care and 27.5% for home- and community-based services (Special Committee on Aging, 2002). This bias does not reflect the preferences of older persons or the fact that many may be able to remain in their homes with a much less intensive amount of care.

However, as states continue to wrestle with aging populations and expanding Medicaid expenditures along with budget reductions, they have begun many experiments in community-based care that serve as alternatives to institutionalization. Several factors, including economics, the preferences of older persons, and the Olmstead Decision—requiring that persons be cared for in the community if they desire and if such care is available—are among the motivating factors for further development of community care. States have begun using a variety of funding sources to expand community care options for older persons. As these continue to be developed and evaluated, they may offer models for replication, resulting in more care options for seniors.

A major challenge in effectively addressing community care needs of older persons is developing the appropriate framework for discerning such needs. A continuing impediment to meeting many care issues is the emphasis placed on physical functioning as the primary criterion for receiving services. Cognitive impairment, mental illness, social resources, and the environment in which the person lives are among the many other factors contributing to assistance needs. However, it is only when these problems are associated with functional impairments that eligibility for community care can be most assured. This myopic perspective focusing on physical functioning means that many older persons are vulnerable to not receiving adequate supports. In addition, timely interventions that might prevent deterioration in functioning may not be available.

Because functional impairments are associated with frailty and incapacity, impaired older persons risk losing their rights to individual autonomy and self-determination. Perspectives that stress the values of beneficence and paternalism can easily threaten choices available to the older person. In these instances they are perceived as being unable to adequately assess their own needs for care or services.

Cash and counseling programs give older persons the right to determine and govern their own care. They counteract negative perceptions by empowering the older person. These programs can play critical roles in expanding community care options by reinforcing the resiliency and ability of the older population. At the same time, safeguards within the programs can help to assure their effectiveness.

Comprehensive instruments to assess individual competency in decisions about and supervision of personal care should be required. In addition, having backup supports available in case the care plan fails could act as further program reinforcement. The challenge in consumer-directed care is balancing ability and autonomy with vulnerability. Educating persons about consumer-directed care and assuring that they understand their own responsibilities and those of the care provider further strengthens the role of these programs.

A major challenge in the recognition and meeting of the needs of seniors is the dearth of professionals and paraprofessionals trained in geriatric care. Some new initiatives aim to add to this workforce by increasing funding for gerontological education and training, and making direct care more attractive to home-care workers. As the population continues to age, with concomitant needs for care, it may also be necessary to focus efforts on changing stereotypes and biases regarding older persons and the aging process. As long as aging is perceived negatively, recruiting the necessary workforce will remain difficult.

Another important challenge is addressing the living environments of older persons for compatibility with their needs. Rather than their having to move to another residence or institution, programs should be provided to enable lower and moderate income persons to modify their own homes. Redesigning existing housing to compensate for difficulties in functioning, and new forms of assistive technology enabling persons to better care for themselves are among services that can make the home livable and reduce the risk of unnecessary institutionalization.

For those having to move to a site that provides more intensive care, assisted living may serve as the most appropriate option. Less restrictive than nursing homes but offering more support services than may be available in one's own home, assisted living offers an important option for many persons with limited functioning. As the housing continues to expand across the country, it should be made more available to those with limited incomes. Currently, the majority of residents pay privately for the housing, with Medicaid covering only a small proportion of residents. Expanding the availability of these facilities to all income groups, while assuring careful regulation and quality care, can make them a truly viable option for many more older persons.

A commitment by the government to the development of more supportive senior public housing is essential. The demand for Section 202 housing far outweighs the supply; yet such housing could play a major role in helping persons to remain in the community. Other government programs, such as the Congregate Housing Services Program and Project Hope, have been found to effectively meet needs of frail older persons in the community and should be expanded. In order to best meet the needs of older persons with impairments, housing and care services must be coordinated.

In order to live comfortably in the community, older persons needing care require a wide array of services. Respite for family caregivers, day care, home care, meals programs, and transportation can be particularly critical in enabling persons to remain in the community. However, a continued shortage of resources prevents these programs from universal availability. Others, who could afford to pay privately for the services, are often unaware of their existence or unsure of how they would meet their needs. By increasing the availability of these important support services more individuals may be able to remain at home. In addition, it is essential to older persons that they and their families be educated and informed about these services so that they may use them, as their care requires.

Long-term care insurance does provide persons with options for home- and community-based services such as home care, assisted living, day care, and respite care. As such it has the potential of increasing the availability of care to many. However, this potential remains limited due to the restricted accessibility of most policies.

Costs place long-term care insurance beyond the means of most persons, with the premiums becoming highest when needs are greatest and income likely to be lower. At the same time, these policies could help reduce persons' dependence on the public sector for assistance, while providing more care options. Making policies more affordable and attractive to younger working persons could help to assure fewer assistance demands on the government, and also provide users with greater flexibility in deciding how their needs for care will be met.

Families continue to provide the bulwark of care to older persons, yet assistance to families remains limited. In fact, it is families themselves that remain challenged by meeting their own needs as caregivers and those of their older relatives. Although the government has begun recognizing these caregivers through income tax credits, family leave, and the Older Americans Act, these programs play only limited roles as support systems.

Traditional values and beliefs underscore the view that families should look after their own with little government interference. This perspective is manifested by government's reluctance to interfere or intrude in caregiver support, which can be conceived as a very private sphere. Such beliefs are bolstered by the fear that with formal interventions, family supports will decrease, therefore increasing the demand for formal services.

Supports through public programs remain limited for family caregivers and are unaffordable to the majority. With the exception of certain state programs, it is questionable that supports provide sufficient amounts of assistance or the options that caregivers need. Many family caregivers are only able to obtain assistance when caregiving has reached a stage of crisis that threatens their continuation in the caregiver role.

Elderly spouses remain at particular risk in their roles as caregivers. Often their own age and physical conditions affect their ability to provide assistance, while their assets and income may make them ineligible for Medicaid support. In addition, their own adherence to norms stressing spousal responsibility and obligations may further deter them from seeking assistance. An absence of information and poor referral systems leave the needs of many of these persons unnoticed. Without appropriate support, these caregivers remain as vulnerable as the persons for whom they are providing care.

Employed caregivers continue to wrestle with the demands of employment and those of their relatives. Although the Family and Medical Leave Act has permitted many to take time from jobs to care for a sick relative, many others continue to be employed by firms not covered by the legislation or who cannot afford to take unpaid leave. A major challenge in meeting the needs of employed caregivers is offering a more extensive program, with leave periods that do not pose a financial hardship. Although such a goal may appear immense, it must be balanced against the huge economic loss that could occur if persons are forced to give up their employment.

Ethnic minority groups face their own challenges as they age. Histories of discrimination, poor services, and inadequate care result in increased risk of impairment and chronic disease. Moreover, the same barriers impeding their service use in their younger years are likely to continue affecting them as they age and require more assistance. In addition, service utilization is dependent upon knowledgeability about a program, and understanding how it can be of assistance.

It is important to recognize that a lack of utilization does not reflect a lack of need. When services are sensitively designed and offered to be compatible with a specific population, they are used. Beliefs that ethnic families are able to care for their own without outside assistance are not acceptable reasons for not offering services. Ethnic caregivers face the same problems and burdens as other families and often with many fewer resources. Assistive interventions are often urgently needed and will be used if offered in a culturally appropriate manner.

As the aging population becomes increasingly diverse, a primary challenge is to rectify past disparities and assure equal access for all groups. This requires knowledgeable and sensitive policy makers and practitioners who understand the ways persons may perceive need and types of assistance. Cultural competency in the design of services helps ensure their compatibility with the values and traditions of specific groups. Models for such programs are in place throughout the country.

Efforts must be made to recognize successful programs so that replication can occur.

As discussed earlier in the book, innovations in community care are occurring in programs and services throughout the country, encouraged by both government and foundation support. States are developing pilot projects, using both Medicare and Medicaid funds, that offer single entry points for services, coordinated institutional and community care, and even the transferring of persons from nursing homes back to the community. Fundamental to many of these programs are coordinated rather than fragmented systems of care, comprehensive services, and knowledge of local needs and priorities. The continued funding and support of such model programs is essential for development of new and creative responses to senior care needs.

Responding to the care needs of an aging society requires flexibility and options, guaranteeing all older persons access to appropriate and desired services. Institutional care will no longer be the most viable measure for providing assistance, due to the sheer growth of the older population. States are beginning to recognize this. Future cohorts of older persons will be better educated, with more resources, and can be expected to demand higher-quality services as long-term care consumers (Stone, 2000). Starting system changes early in the 21st century would benefit today's older population, as well as aid in preventing a crisis when the demands of 77 million baby boomers are felt.

New opportunities for the development of services are beginning and policy makers will need to begin making decisions about their future growth and forms. The impetus for change is already present: The economic realities of the current system, with its dependence on institutional care, have been noticeably felt in state budgets. Thus, although much of the motivation to develop home- and community-based care may stem more from economic than humanitarian concerns, the impetus is there. The challenge now is not only maintaining but strengthening this focus, so that an aging society becomes a comfortable and secure place for present and future generations of older persons. Models and care innovations exist, but until their implementation becomes a national priority, community care will remain a concept rather than a reality for the majority of Americans.

REFERENCES

Collopy, B. (1988). Autonomy in long-term care: Some crucial distinctions. *Gerontologist, 28* (Supplement), 10–17.

Special Committee on Aging, U.S. Senate. (2002, June). *Hearing finding summary.* Washington, DC: U.S. Government Printing Office.

Stone, R. (2000). *Long-term care for the elderly with disabilities: Current policy, emerging trends, and implications for the 21st century.* New York: Milbank Memorial Fund.

Index

Springer Publishing Company

Multidisciplinary Perspectives on Aging

Lynn M. Tepper, MA, MS, EDM, EdD
Thomas M. Cassidy, MA, Editors

In this multidisciplinary text, noted leaders from a variety of fields provide students and professionals with a big picture approach to the best possible care for today's growing aging population. Addressing the extensive concerns that have arisen out of an increased life expectancy and the "elder-boom" of aging baby boomers, the contributors point to changing care and housing needs; health, mental health, and wellness c o n-cerns; and financial, ethical, and legal issues in elder care.

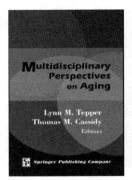

Partial Contents:

Part I: Changing Relationships, Changing Care Needs • Aging in America: Challenges and Opportunities, *L.M. Tepper, MA, MS, EdM, EdD* • Family Relationships and Support Networks, *L.M. Tepper, MA, MS,EdM, EdD* • The Nursing Home and the Continuum of Care, *W.T. Smith, MSW, PhD* • Environmental Design in Evoking the Capacities of Older People, *L.G. Hiatt, PhD* • Avoiding Institutional Care: The Home Health Care Option, *C. DeLorey, RN, MPH, PhD*

Part II: Health and Wellness in Later Life • Medical Care of the Elderly, *R.H. Rubin, MD, FACP* • Health Promotion in Later Life, *C. Kopes-Kerr, MD* • Considerations for Oral Health in the Elderly, *B.M. Horrell, DDS, MS* • Major Mental Disorders of Old Age, *G.J. Kennedy, MD* • Counseling Older People and Their Families, *L.M. Tepper, MA, MS,EdM, EdD*

Part III: Financial, Ethical, and Legal Issues in Elder Care End-of Life Issues from a Social Service Perspective, *S.S. Robinson, LMSW, PhD and L.M. Tepper, MA, MS,EdM, EdD* • Financing Health Care, *T.C. Jackson, MPH, CEBS* • Elder Law, *M.B. Kapp, JD, MPH, FCLM* • Elder Ethics, *E.R. Chichin, PhD, RN* • Identifying and Preventing Elder Abuse, *T.M. Cassidy, MA* • Interdisciplinary Teamwork: The Key to Quality Care for Older Adults, *P.A. Miller, EdD, OTR, FAOTA*

2004   304pp   0-8261-1734-1   hard

11 West 42nd Street, New York, NY 10036-8002 • Fax: 212-941-7842
Order Toll-Free: 877-687-7476 • Order On-line: www.springerpub.com